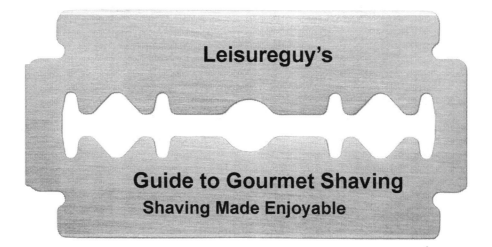

Leisureguy's

Guide to Gourmet Shaving
Shaving Made Enjoyable

Sixth Edition

By
Michael Ham
'Leisureguy'

Pogonotomy Press
Monterey California

Edition 6.0 – August 2012
ISBN 978-1477436806

To EH, who has found it useful
To GM and CM and BH, who someday will read it
To KV, for the phrase "gourmet shaving"
To K★, for taking up wetshaving
And, of course, to The Wife, for listening to all these
discoveries with exemplary forbearance.

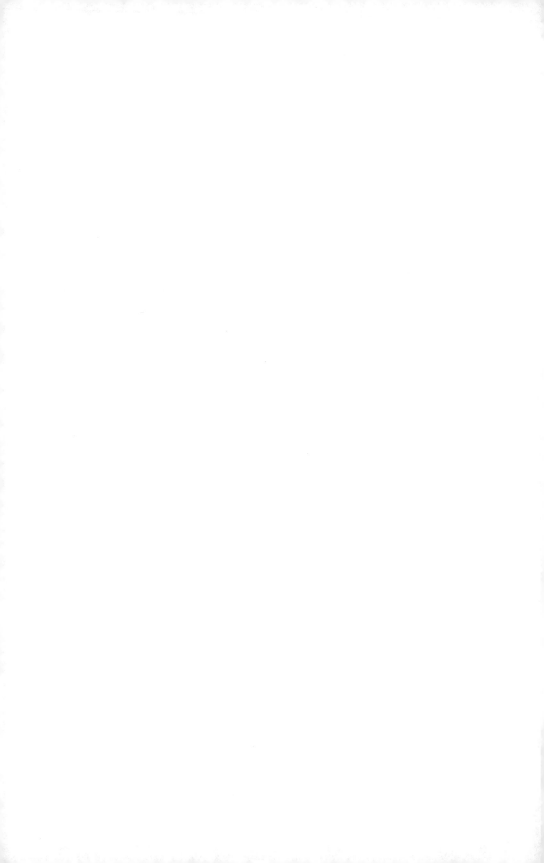

Contents

Preface to the Sixth Edition

I REALIZED recently that this book might have been more accurately titled *The Epicure's Guide to Shaving*, for Epicurus[1] would surely approve making necessary tasks enjoyable. He thought that chance encounters of atoms falling through the void, randomly interacting, produced—after much time—us and the world in which we live. In his view we cease to exist when we die, while the atoms continue their tumbling journey through time and space.

Because Epicurus believed that life is a one-shot deal, enjoying life has a high priority. A dissolute lifestyle tends to have highly unpleasant consequences, so it makes sense to seek enjoyment first in the small things of life, which is what we mostly encounter day to day. Learning new ideas and mastering new skills are examples of activities that provide enjoyment without harm.

Take, as a random example, the morning shave: an Epicurean who shaves will look for a way to derive enjoyment from the task: to spend his (limited) time doing things he doesn't enjoy makes no sense when he could instead do them enjoyably. Moreover, when a task is enjoyable, doing it requires no willpower: you are drawn to the task rather than having to push yourself. Indeed, a task can even be restorative and energizing; rather than draining you, the task approached properly can provide both enjoyment a sense of fulfillment.

The psychologist Mihály Csíkszentmihályi wrote several books on a mental state he termed "flow": a focused, absorbing, satisfying involvement in what is happening in the moment[2]. So another way to state the Epicurean position is that one should arrange his or her life to maximize the opportunities for flow to occur. Flow is a mental experience, so introspection combined with an attitude that encourages the enjoyment of small things—to *look* for joy, and to think about how to find more occasions of joy—is an obvious step.

This book is my contribution to an Epicurean lifestyle: the book offers a way to make a necessary chore enjoyable. But don't stop with just shaving.

I note that traditional wetshaving continues to grow rapidly:

- New on-line vendors of traditional shaving products continue to appear. The vendor list now has well over 100 entries.
- On-line forums devoted to shaving continue to increase in number and in membership. Reddit's Wicked_Edge grew from 3,000 members six months ago to 16,000 as I write—and is still growing rapidly.

- Not only are established manufacturers introducing new safety razors, we're also seeing *new* manufacturers: iKon, Tradere, and Weber, for example, make top-quality razors. I wrote an article in Sharpologist about the implications of this phenomenon[3].
- The prices of vintage safety razors on eBay continue to increase, which indicates that demand continues to increase.

All this is evidence that the number of men who have decided abandon expensive, heavily advertised shaving tools for the pleasures and comfort of traditional shaving is growing rapidly. I hope you'll join us.

Although the total number of traditional wetshaving vendors has increased, some vendors have closed their doors since the previous edition. Many of the vendors mentioned in the Appendix are small operations that depend totally on one or two people. Naturally enough, such businesses are vulnerable to disruption or sudden shutdown from any number of causes: health problems or the passing of the proprietor or a family member, or financial exigencies (or the opposite: the fine on-line store Razor and Brush had to close when its owner, who ran the business as a sideline, was promoted to a more demanding job), or for other reasons.

These businesses, which often offer exceptional handcrafted products of high quality, have a certain cherry-blossom quality: they bloom briefly and their products may be available only for a relatively short time. I now treasure irreplaceable soaps, creams, and equipment that I purchased only a few years ago from businesses now gone, never to return.

If you like any products offered by these artisans and small-business owners, buy promptly. You will get something that you can use and enjoy, possibly long after the business is gone. Shop early and often and stock up for your future needs—and when you're thinking about gifts, consider how a good brush and a shaving soap or shaving cream can improve anyone's shave.

I thank AM, who kept after me until I wrote this book, and thanks as well to the shavers who have suggested ideas and improvements for the book. Special thanks to betelgeux, cathartica, greyzer, HeyRememberThatTime, mpperry, Dirty Texan, Hyzerflip, NoHelmet, psywiped, wicked_VD, do_not_follow, Release-the-Kraken, JustHereForTheTips, and others of the Wicked_Edge community for their insights and interest. They have increased my understanding with their questions (especially those from newbies) and their discoveries.

Michael Ham
Monterey, California
gourmetshaving@gmail.com

Preface

FOR most men, shaving is a daily yet unappealing task: a routine at best, and more often a tedious, boring, hateful chore. A surprising number of men believe that they have "sensitive skin" because the tug-and-cut action of the common multiblade shaving cartridge and the pressure these men exert on the razor trying to get a close shave, together with inadequate beard preparation from a pressurized can of dry, foamy shaving mix and a tendency to use the cartridge well beyond its useful life (because of the cost of replacing it), produces skin irritation, razor burn, razor bumps, and in-grown hairs.

You can avoid all that: the daily shaving task can easily be transformed into a pleasurable ritual that leaves the shaver feeling renewed and pampered and his skin healthy. All it takes are the right tools and a little practice.

This book introduces the shaver to the world of traditional wetshaving: the shaving brush, exquisitely formulated shaving soaps and creams, and well-designed safety razors—readily available and still being manufactured—that use a double-edged blade to provide a smooth (and enjoyable) shave.

Moreover, the blades (which usually last a week) are much cheaper than cartridges—even if the shaver continues to use his cartridges beyond their effective lifespan (to postpone the expense of replacing them).

The learning curve is short and the enjoyment immense, so start today. You can jump to the section on the recommended beginner's kit, but I suggest you first read through the book: as always is the case, your choice of equipment requires balancing various tradeoffs, and you may be unfamiliar with those involved in wetshaving.

A shave, like Gaul, is divided into three parts:

1. **Prep** – Preparation is everything you do before picking up the razor. Prep usually involves first a shower, and then at the sink a pre-shave soap, a shaving brush, and shaving cream or shaving soap.
2. **Shave** – Once prep is complete, you pick up the razor and shave; this step involves only the razor and the blade (which is not so simple as you think, as you'll learn later) with a focus on pressure and angle.
3. **Aftershave** – Once you rinse and put away the razor, you do the final steps, generally involving an alum block and an aftershave and

occasionally, should you get a nick, a styptic. Aftershaves come in many forms (splashes, balms, creams, gels, etc.), and your choice of aftershave may vary with the season if you live where winter's cold.

In explaining how to shave I shall follow the above sequence, discussing the tools and techniques appropriate to each step. (You'll also find a chapter on skin issues—acne, razor bumps, ingrowns, dry skin, and so on.) Before beginning the shave, however, I'll provide some background to establish the context.

Note that you may want to move to traditional wetshaving in two steps. With Step 1 you master prep, as described above, but continue to use your cartridge razor. You learn the grain of your beard and how to prepare it for a good shave—this in itself will greatly improve your shave. Then later, once that is in hand, you take Step 2: get double-edged blades and a safety razor and learn to use those. (Some readers may even want to take a third step: to get a straight razor and master that kind of shave. I include a brief section on taking that step, but straight-razor shaving is not the subject of this book.)

Men on a student budget will immediately see that this two-step approach splits the cost into two small purchases instead of one bigger one: Step 1 can come from one month's paycheck and Step 2 from the following month's. Moreover, the two-step approach means the novice shaver has to learn only one set of skills at a time: first prep, then shaving. The chapter "Recommendations for a beginner" thus uses this two-step approach.

This book is the culmination of much experimentation and trial-and-error, along with many suggestions and contributions from others. All quotations are, of course, used with the permission of the authors, and I hope their insights help you as they have helped me.

ONE

What this is

THIS book is for men who shave without enjoyment or who are just learning to shave. It describes a method of shaving that transforms a daily chore into a pleasurable ritual. It's a beginner's guide to wetshaving: how to shave with a safety razor and not hurt yourself. (A safety razor uses a double-edged blade and is often called a "DE razor.")

Shaving with a safety razor and using a shaving brush and high-quality shaving cream or soap for lather has several benefits:

- The shave itself is enjoyable and satisfying.
- Your skin feels better because a double-edged blade cuts the whiskers easily and cleanly, unlike electric razors and the "tug-and-cut" action of the multiblade disposable cartridge (which also encourages in-growns).
- The cost of shaving is substantially less. Double-edged blades cost pennies and are normally good for 4-6 shaves; a puck of shaving soap or tub of shaving cream lasts for months.
- You get a smoother, closer shave without irritating your skin.

This guide takes you step by step through the process. It discusses in detail the equipment and supplies you need and where to get them and, for the do-it-yourselfer, how to make some yourself. It describes how to prepare your beard for a shave and the basic techniques in building a good lather and using the razor. It provides guidance for dealing with common problems like acne and razor bumps. And it points to on-line sources of more information that can help you address any particular problems you might encounter.

My goal is to provide the novice safety-razor shaver with a useful and comprehensive reference that provides answers not only to the questions he has but also to questions he didn't know to ask. Based on the feedback and comments I've received, that goal has been achieved.

I should note that I am a "shave critic," and my recommendations, like those of a movie critic or restaurant critic, are based on my own direct experience. I buy products as a regular customer, at retail, and I receive no remuneration, kickbacks, discounts, or other consideration from manufacturers or dealers. I retain my independence and maintain an arm's-length relationship with vendors (whom I like, admire, and respect) so that I will not feel I have to tailor my opinions to curry favor or repay special treatment. What you read in this book is simply what it appears to be: an independent assessment from a man who enjoys a good shave with proper tools and fine products.

Companion web page

The Web is home to a vast profusion of information about almost any topic, including shaving. In no way could I include in this book all the information—much of it useful—that you can find on the Web. But, I realized, I can provide *links* to some of that information.

So my approach to writing the book was to include in the book all the essential information to take you into the pleasures of shaving with brush and soap and safety razor—and also to provide links to ancillary information that you may find interesting and/or useful. My suggestion is that you simply read the book, reserving the links for later, and only for those things that you want to explore further.

To improve the readability of the text—and because I suggest that you start by simply reading the book without looking up all the links—I've placed the links in endnotes following the Appendix. And, to make the links even easier to use, I've also provided them on the Web as hyperlinks so that you can simply click each to go to the site of interest.

The companion Web page listing the links is especially worth checking since I update it as new information becomes available—for example, price changes that affect recommendations, or the appearance of new vendors or products. See **tinyurl.com/leisureguy6** for the list of clickable links. I recommend that you bookmark that page.

You can review shaving posts on leisureguy.wordpress.com (my blog) by clicking "shaving" in Category Search. That will present all shaving entries in abbreviated form—click on the title of any post to see the whole thing. If you comment on a post, I will normally reply. Links to some specific shaving posts can be found on the "Useful Posts" page of the blog (see the list of links at the right when viewing the blog).

TWO

Who I am and why this book

I BEGAN shaving (with a Gillette DE safety razor) around 1955. Then I switched to a Schick Injector, a safety razor that uses a single-edged blade. But that was then, in the dark ages of the isolated shaver, when each shaver had to depend on his own knowledge and what he could pick up from his family and friends.

The only sources of information I had, for example, were my step-dad (who knew no more than I about shaving) and commercials and ads, whose general content was, "Buy this product." I used a brush, Old Spice shaving soap, and Gillette Blue Blades, and my shave consisted of two complete passes: one down, and one up, the second pass without lather. I used little pieces of toilet paper on the resulting nicks and over the course of my high-school career must have used up several rolls. As soon as I got to college, I grew a beard.

I still remember reading in high school a near-future science-fiction novel about a guy getting ready for a big night. He lathers up and shaves with the grain, then he lathers up *again* and shaves against the grain. I thought, "That's odd—he lathered a *second* time." It never occurred to me that lathering before each pass might be the right way to shave.

Today—now—is truly the golden age of shaving. Only with the Internet has it been possible for the far-flung band of safety-razor shavers to pool the knowledge gained from their experience and trials and provide all shavers, new or old, with so much information, and to gain easy access to vendors of wet-shaving products all over the globe.

This book grew out of my own experience, augmented and illuminated by experiences and questions other shavers posted in the on-line shaving forums. I thank the guys on the shaving forums, particularly ShaveNook.com and Reddit's Wicked_Edge. I also thank the vendors listed in the appendix for the fine array of products and information they offer, essential to the practice of traditional shaving. And in particular I want to thank shaving novices, whose questions and desire for a reliable and organized introduction to wetshaving first stimulated this book.

I am not a dermatologist or a cosmetologist and have no professional background in skin care or shaving. I am a retired guy who found a way to make shaving enjoyable, and I wrote this book as a report of my own experience and observations, not as recommendations specific to you, whom I don't know. My hope is that you will find in it tools and techniques you can adapt to your own situation, at your own pleasure and risk. I certainly cannot guarantee the results, since I don't know what your shaving issues might be. So read, enjoy, be judicious in your experimentation, and observe outcomes closely.

With the existence of the Internet and active shaving forums, is a book like this even needed? I believe it is. For one thing, a book, unlike a collection of Internet links, can serve as a gift for men who hate to shave, and I hope that this volume will often be among presents such men receive for graduation, Father's Day, bar mitzvahs, birthdays, and other gift occasions—most especially those men for whom shaving is still an unrewarding chore.

Some who receive the book will not have previously considered traditional wetshaving. One of their friends or family members knew that they found shaving a tedious, hateful task and gave them the book so they could *enjoy* the morning shave. Thus the next chapter makes the case for traditional wetshaving—just in case you're now considering the idea for the first time.

Although the Internet does provide access to much information, that information is disorganized and inconsistent, so a beginning shaver must spend considerable time wading through esoteric minutiae discussed at length while searching for basic guidance—fundamental information that may be hidden, glossed over, misstated, or omitted altogether (because "everyone already knows that"). Of course, beginners can ask questions in shaving forums, but newbies often don't know what questions to ask and sometimes fear to expose their ignorance. This book was written for a beginning shaver who values his time and wants an organized and consistent presentation of reliable information.

Information in online shaving forums also is volatile: new threads constantly push old threads out of sight, and occasionally entire threads are deleted, erasing all the information and photos they once contained. The information in this book will still be here when you return.

The shaving forums are nonetheless valuable, and I encourage you to participate. For one thing, you can ask questions about specific problems that you encounter (and the final chapter includes a useful template for getting information efficiently). For another, it is through the forums that word quickly spreads of new products and new ideas. Also, questions asked there can stir your thinking and lead to new approaches. I learned much, subjecting it to my own judgment, tests, and interpretation, and made some discoveries of my own.

I hope that this book will be an enjoyable and informative companion in your journey of exploration.

THREE

Why to do it

BEFORE we start, I should answer the question, "Why bother?" Why put aside all the modern technology of pressurized cans of shaving foams and gels and the modern multiblade razor cartridge that allows you to shave while still half asleep? Why pick up tools and techniques from a generation (or two) ago? Traditional shavers offer several answers.

Care of skin

Some reasons to switch to traditional wetshaving are pragmatic and down-to-earth: the multiblade cartridge uses a tug-and-cut technique that, combined with the dry chemical foam squirted from a pressurized can and the pressure required to pull 3, 4, 5, or 6 blades at a time through stubble, leads to ingrown whiskers, razor bumps, and skin irritation. Many shavers who experience these problems think that they have "sensitive skin." They continue to suffer, buying loads of products promoted as protective pre-shaves or as soothing and healing aftershaves in hopes of repairing the damage. Some, however, switch to the double-edged blade and safety razor and find that, after mastering the techniques and skills of traditional shaving, their skin problems disappear.

This seems counterintuitive. Shaving has been a part of human culture from very early in our development—even some stone-age humans had razors of obsidian, which can be substantially sharper than a modern steel razor[4] as modern anthropologists (and straight razor shavers) who have tried obsidian blades for shaving have found[5]. With such a long period of development, one would think that the most modern and recently designed shaving tools would be the best, but marketing has the power to cloud men's minds (and, alas, has never pledged to use its power only for good). The marketing of shaving tools nowadays is much better and more effective than the shaving tools themselves[6].

I repeatedly read shaving-forum posts by guys with bad skin conditions—acne, for example, or razor bumps—that clear up shortly after they begin shaving with a DE cartridge. It's so noticeable a trend that an experiment is in order. If you're a cartridge shaver, and you have skin problems, particularly if they seem microbe-related, try switching to traditional wetshaving with a DE razor and see whether the problem clears. The cost is not high: Bruce Everiss described a low-cost, high-luxury shave kit[7] that you can assemble for around $45—the cost of a dozen Fusion cartridges. The Frank Shaving brush is permanent, and the soap stick lasts a long time. Even less costly: the Omega 11047 boar/badger brush (less than $20), a terrific little brush, and a tube of Speick shaving cream ($6 or so), and quite often you can find a vintage DE safety razor for free (from a family member who once shaved that way) or for a pittance at a garage sale, thrift shop, flea market, or the like. Whipped Dog offers a beginner kit that runs $31[8].

One reason so many cartridge shavers believe they have sensitive skin is that cartridges now have high blade counts (3-6 blades). As a result, the shaver must force the razor to cut through 3-6 blades' worth of stubble at once. It requires noticeable effort to pull that many blades simultaneously through stubble even when the blades are sharp. And because cartridges are so expensive, many shavers continue using them long after the edges are worn dull—stropping cartridges on denim to eke out a few more shaves is a common practice. (Cartridge blades are made from the same steel as DE blades, and DE blades generally last only about a week before the edge dulls and the blade begins to tug and pull as it cuts and so is replaced.)

The effort needed to pull multiple blades through the stubble explains why cartridge shavers, after their first shave with a DE safety razor, often comment on how *easy* it is: "It's no effort at all! It just *glides* along!" Sure: they are now using a razor that cuts only one blade's worth of stubble at a time: much less resistance from stubble, resulting in a much easier shave with little pressure required—generally just the weight of the razor.

Moreover, to keep the blade in contact with the skin when pulling a cartridge with so much force requires a lot of pressure *against* the skin. So the cartridge shaver presses hard, scraping his skin with 3-6 blades at a time, most of the time after the blades have dulled from use.

Force and pressure mash stubble, foam, and flakes of skin into the crevices, nooks, and crannies of the cartridge's moist, dark interior. Result: a microbe incubator, and often the shaver's face breaks out after shaving. A DE safety razor has fewer places for microbes to linger and easily rinses clean, so such skin problem often vanish as soon as a shaver makes the switch to DE.

If pimples appear after you shave with a multiblade cartridge, try this: after finishing the shave, first rinse your cartridge razor head well under hot water and then rinse it in high-proof (70% or higher) rubbing alcohol. And before starting your shave, rinse the razor head again in the rubbing alcohol. Also try using a fresh shaving towel daily—thin, lint-free barber towels (also known as bar towels) cost about $11/dozen and are easy to launder. Or just switch to a DE razor. Once you switch to traditional wetshaving tools and methods, you will likely notice that your skin becomes clearer and healthier.

A guy in one of the shaving forums commented that he started traditional shaving and, after a few months, returned home from college to see his mom. She felt his cheek and commented that it was the smoothest and softest it had been since he was 5. He said he had been aware that traditional shaving had improved his skin, but the improvement was so gradual he really didn't understand how dramatic the change was.[9]

Quality of shave

A "good shave" is of course smooth and without razor burn, irritation, nicks or cuts—but that's merely the absolute minimum, and any shave that doesn't rise to that level is not worth considering. Beyond that, a good shave must be *enjoyable*: it should not merely produce a good outcome, but the experience itself must be a pleasure. Otherwise, what's the point? To toe the line to satisfy grooming conventions, getting nothing out of it for yourself? That's the sad lot of too many.

Men who choose a safety razor with a double-edged blade find they get a better shave, one that's smoother, closer, and longer-lasting. This contradicts ads about the latest disposable multiblade cartridges, but ads—brace yourself—frequently stretch the truth. Guys who have switched from cartridge to DE safety razors fairly often say that their kids or grandkids comment that their face is not so scratchy as it used to be. They find that a traditional shave has a smoother result than a cartridge shave.

In fact, the very closest shaves are probably done with a skillfully wielded straight razor, but using a straight razor demands a panoply of skills, including honing and stropping. This book focuses on the DE razor, which uses an inexpensive, disposable, double-edged blade.

Cost of shave

As I write this, one Gillette Fusion ProGlide disposable multiblade cartridge costs $3.64 (Amazon discount price for pack of 8). One double-edged blade, which will normally last a week (depending on brand of blade and nature of beard), generally costs around 25¢ but better prices are available with bulk purchases. As I write, Derby blades are available for $12.93/200, so that a shaver who likes Derbies can shave for a *year* and spend just $3.37 for blades. (In fairness, the Derby brand doesn't work for everyone—as discussed in the chapter on blades. My own best brand costs 9¢ per blade compared to 6.5¢ for Derbys.)

Gillette claims that a cartridge lasts for five weeks of shaving[10] (although cartridge shavers agree that after the first week or two the comfort level drops significantly), so during those 45 weeks the ~~poor sap~~ cartridge shaver will buy 9 cartridges (5 weeks each for 45 weeks), for a total cost of $32.76. That's **ten** times the cost of Derbys—*if* the five-week figure is not some advertising fantasy.

Given the price, some cartridge shavers gamely continue to use the same cartridge for three months or more. In that scenario, the suffering shaver will buy four cartridges a year: $14.56, about four times the cost of the DE blades.

For lather, a puck of shaving soap—say, one from Honeybee Soaps—costs less than $5 and in daily use will last around 3 months. The razor and the brush last a lifetime—indeed, even longer: some shavers enjoy using double-edged razors from 80 or more years ago.

Andrew Webster built a three-page Excel workbook for a detailed cost analysis of your shave, both for multiblade cartridges with canned foam and for traditional wetshaving with brush, soap, and DE razor and blades[11]. It contains costs, number of shaves per container (of soaps, shaving creams, aftershaves, and the like), and product ratings. Alter his entries to match your own choices, costs, and ratings. Treat the figures in the workbook as "illustrations" because (for example) the number of shaves per soap varies greatly by shaver due to shaving technique, water hardness, and the like. Enter your own data and use the workbook to analyze those to find your own cost savings and breakeven point.

Quality of life

"Quality of life" refers both to the quality of one's own personal life and also to the quality of the environment in which we all live.

Environmental benefits

The environmental benefits of traditional wetshaving are obvious: the landfill impact is negligible, and soap and shaving cream are benign. A year of shaving with a DE safety razor uses about 50 double-edged blades and their paper wrappers and a puck of shaving soap (a triple-milled soap may well last a year). In contrast, using a cartridge system means discarding a dozen (or more) plastic and metal cartridges, the plastic packaging in which they come, and several cans that formerly contained pressurized shaving foam. For my discarded blades—

which are recyclable since they are pure metal—I use a small can that once held evaporated milk: after six years it is only now becoming filled.

In terms of environmental impact, there's no comparison. Indeed, even a comparison of ingredients between a can of shaving foam and a puck of shaving soap will show that the soap is more environment-friendly (and, one imagines, kinder to the skin).

Personal benefits

I didn't have skin problems and wasn't all that unhappy with the shaves the Mach 3 delivered. I turned to safety-razor shaving for the sheer pleasure the morning shave now provides. Shaving has changed from a routine at best, a chore more often, to a wonderful ritual from which I emerge feeling truly pampered. I now *look forward* to shaving each day. That feeling more than repays the little bit of equipment required. The daily shave: a daily pleasure. How many men can say that?

Very few. I suspect that the current fashion of young men wearing a stubble of 4 or 5 days' growth originated because shaving is unpleasant for most men who use today's shaving paraphernalia. Fashion photographers, seeing many young men with visible stubble, decided it was a "look," and put such men in ads, trying to appeal to that demographic. In fact, these young men simply don't like to shave but for whatever reason may not grow a full beard. So they put off shaving, and the look becomes a fashion statement that means their Significant Other gets a sandpaper experience with every kiss.

Those who use traditional equipment, in sharp contrast, *enjoy* shaving. Indeed, the focused attention and meditative mindset of shaving with a safety razor can provide a morning ritual not unlike the Zen tea ceremony:

Special room – check
Special mode of dress – check
Contemplative, unrushed mindset – check
Cleanliness and order – check
Practice of technique requires focused attention (aka flow) – check
Use of special tools, often old – check
Tools both functional and aesthetically pleasing – check
Suspension of mind chatter, critical judgments – check
Senses—sight, hearing, touch, smell—fully engaged – check
Physical enjoyment of sources of warmth – check
Awareness & enjoyment of aromas arising from hot water – check
Definite sequence of steps – check
Structure of the entire experience repeated each time – check
Feeling of pleasure, fulfillment, and satisfaction at end - check

In the preface I mentioned the mental state of "flow," in which one loses consciousness of self and of time, becoming totally focused on a task whose intricacy and difficulty require about 85% of one's capacity. (Attention wanders when a task is too easy, and if it's too difficult, anxiety disrupts flow and reduces enjoyment.)

Most people know from their own experience that a state of happiness is usually recognized only after the fact—at the time, one is unaware of it *per se*, but simply enjoys each moment. Flow seems to exactly describe the state of experiencing happiness, so the more flow one can arrange, the happier one's life. Shaving, with the right approach and mindset and attention, can promote flow.

The contemplative aspect of a satisfying shaving ritual is revitalizing. Most of us live hurried lives, multitasking and rushing about, harried by time demands. What the morning shave with a safety razor offers is a small oasis of unhurried calm and single-minded attention to remind you what it feels like to be unrushed and not to be doing one thing while thinking of something else.

The morning shave is not only restorative in itself, it provides a foundation of structure for the morning: men who once leapt from bed, quickly ran a cartridge razor over their beard (or skipped a day), took a quick bite of breakfast, and went out the door, lurching into the day's events off-balance, find with wetshaving that they instead develop an entire morning sequence, ordered and satisfying, that provides a stable platform from which to launch the day.

And modern psychology even suggests that this shaving ritual can increase your self-esteem: Cognitive dissonance[12] posits that a person holding contradictory beliefs (or observing himself acting in contradiction to his beliefs) will add to or modify his beliefs to resolve or reduce the contradiction[13].

I thought of this regarding shaving (of course). By acquiring the specialized tools and supplies and taking the time and care to create a shaving ritual, the shaver presents himself with a behavior that leads to increased self-esteem: "If I'm taking this much time to pamper myself, I must be worth it." Not a bad feeling at all. And the cumulative effect of having the feeling reinforced every weekday morning can be substantial, as described by one shaver[14]:

> Throughout my life I have been saddled with responsibility and plunged knee deep into competition, whether it was through my parents' or my own volition. From a very young age competition enveloped me. From my school work, with ever-critical parents pushing me to do better, to whatever sport I was playing at the time, competition was an active and dominating force for me.
>
> During my undergraduate studies, my hobbies eventually focused themselves due to a minimum of time available. My life was consumed with

essentially two main activities: schoolwork and my sport at the time, fencing. My parents' critical nature had worked itself into my persona by this point, and therefore every practice, every competition I went to was filled with self-judgment, stress, and just dwelling on how I screwed up and why I lost. It was not something I could easily just forget about after the fact, but something that constantly lingered.

My studies eventually led me to graduate school, where the competition and stress rose further. As the only white person in my research group, it was made fully aware to me from the beginning that my being white (in a group of Chinese/Taiwanese students) meant that I had all eyes on me, as I was told that because I was white I was automatically assumed as being lazy. Pressure to surpass expectations was high. While I had stopped fencing, I picked up cycling, which led to racing, which led to more intense training and competition. It seems that no matter what I chose it centered on competition. Eventually, I lost the joy of my hobbies, and everything had become a chore, a task, an obstacle to overcome. There was less enjoyment, just stress to do better.

I tried finding some new hobbies, something I could enjoy just for fun. I tried throwing darts again with my buddy, but that led to a weekly darts tournament. I tried picking up golf to play with my girlfriend, but the self-critical nature keeps creeping in with every slice, every topped ball, every trek through the rough, every goddamn water hazard.

After graduate school there was work, which continued to bury me under mountains of stress and anxiety. Combined with hobbies that also seem to promote stress in me, I noticed a complete lack of any outlet for my stress that didn't just generate more. It was bad.

Then I found traditional wetshaving. "What an odd thing," I thought. How could shaving have this many devotees? How could such a chore have so much enthusiasm behind it? Is there a similar group of people who love folding laundry? *What the hell is wrong with these people?* I'd had straight razor shaves before, and they were very nice, but this? This just seemed like too much.

I did my research, I trudged through the volumes of information present here, and eventually picked up my own kit and began the process. Leisureguy really does make an apt analogy in that it's almost like a Japanese tea ceremony and is very Zen-like. Psychologists worldwide will agree that self-reflection, meditation, and general "quiet time" are all needed in order to be healthy, happy, and sane. Up until this point, I never had the ability, or had a reason, to make this time available to me. Suddenly I had the time. The concentration needed for shaving helped me focus, but at the same time I was able to approach it differently than every other hobby. It was not a competition, it was not a race, it was not going to be graded or judged, it was an activity, an action with definite steps to follow, a procedure. I like procedures.

The methodical nature of shaving made for a much-needed routine and regularity in my hectic schedule. A definite time set aside for me. Not for my friends, nor my coworkers, nor my boss, nor my family, nor my lovely and patient girlfriend, but for me. To be able to shut everything and everyone away once a day for a short amount of time and not be questioned as to why I was being withdrawn or reclusive is extremely relaxing. The result? More confidence from learning a new skill and looking better; less stress due to a set schedule, routine, and procedure; enjoyment of a new hobby because I can still tinker (new soaps, blades, etc.); and an overall better outlook on things due to all of the above.

Somehow I have found a hobby, as silly as it might seem to some outside this group, which quite literally makes me feel better about life in general. While it may only be a small part of a bigger picture, it's *my* small part.

I believe that shaving's freedom from stress and competition stems in part from the gradual realization that discovering what works best for you doesn't put you ahead or behind any other shaver—he, too, is engaged in figuring out his own optimal combination. Thus there's no external measure or standard to meet or beat: when shaving, one is totally engaged in achieving the best shave he can for himself: he is very much involved in the particularities of the moment and removed from other worries and concerns that plague us. Our lives indeed consist of these particularities of the present moment. If we can pay attention to them, rather than worrying about the future, obsessing about the past, and measuring ourselves against others, we find ourselves recentered and renewed.

The role that traditional wetshaving can play in personal renewal is something others have commented on[15]. Even though it works at an unconscious level, cognitive dissonance is powerful, and starting each day taking time and care to do something that is clearly for yourself, treating yourself nicely, gradually results in feeling that you must be worth this effort: if you don't feel that, cognitive dissonance results, and the simplest way to resolve it, given that you continue the self-care, is to accept that you deserve it. That means you start to view yourself in a better light, and thus you begin acting in ways consistent with that view—that is, you unconsciously start living up to how you now view yourself, which results in observing yourself doing things that such a person would do, thus reconfirming to yourself that you are indeed this better person, which leads to more good actions to maintain your image as a person you respect, and so on: a virtuous circle.

The fact is that in any situation or circumstance, most people already know what they should do or the decision they should make. (This is evident when people say that don't know what to do in a situation, and when asked what a counselor or a coach or a religious leader or a teacher would advise, they generally can state the advice they would get.)

Starting each day with a ritual of personal grooming adds just enough push so that you do some things and make some decisions that you already know you *should* do or make, and those steps are enough start the cycle of positive feedback, which can grow quickly (cf. regenerative feedback).

This process works because the force driving it is *unobtrusive*—that is, it comes from doing a routine and necessary task—and *enjoyable* (honey draws more flies than does vinegar: people learn faster from seeking pleasure than from avoiding pain) and (quite important) *daily*. The push may be small, but it's steady, and once the effects begin, the process picks up speed because of its self-reinforcing (regenerative) nature.

Moving to a more mundane level: men who suffer from hay fever and other such allergies improve their quality of life by shaving during allergy season. Pollen and other allergens get trapped in mustaches and beards, exacerbating the sneezing and sniffling. To minimize symptoms, men with facial hair should wash it frequently during the day, particularly after being outside— or (easier and simpler) stay clean-shaven during allergy season.

An important quality-of-life consideration for most men is their sex life. Stiff, abrasive stubble is unsuited to the tender intimacies of lovemaking compared to skin that's smooth-shaven and fragrant.

A summary of reasons men enjoy traditional shaving:

- **Sensual enjoyment**: hot lather, the feel of a flexible yet firm shaving brush, the razor making a nice sound as it mows through the stubble, feeling your smooth face after the shave, the fragrances of the lather and the aftershave, etc., as well as the pleasures of making love without abrasive stubble.
- **Flow**: as described above: focused attention on a task that requires around 85% of your capabilities, with a clear goal and immediate feedback as you work at it. It really clears the mind.
- **Gadget appeal**: brush styles, razor mechanisms, blade characteristics, soap varieties, etc.
- The great feeling of **transforming a daily chore into a daily pleasure**: conquering, in a small way, drudgery itself.

- **Frugality**: the satisfaction of knowing that soap and blade cost just pennies, rather than the high-priced products of marketing that other men typically use.
- Finally, **getting the best (smoothest, closest) shaves** of your life with zero skin irritation.

The YMMV factor

A common saying in traditional wetshaving is "YMMV": "Your mileage may vary." The proverb of the same sentiment is "One man's meat is another's poison." In shaving, *nothing* works for *everyone*. (And this principle—like others I shall point out—applies with broader generality than just in shaving.)

Although something—a razor, a blade, a soap, an aftershave—may work extremely well for me, it may not work at all for you. An obvious example: some men have skin sensitive to (for example) sandalwood. Although I may love my sandalwood soap or aftershave, a man who's sensitive to it would find it awful to use. And these are not "right" and "wrong" issues—it is simply that what works for me may not for you, and vice versa: YMMV.

Strangely, the YMMV phenomenon particularly affects blades. One would expect that objective standards of sharpness would rule, but in fact shavers vary tremendously in their responses to any brand of blade: a blade that was a "best blade" for me was termed "a tragic waste of metal" by another shaver. Who was right? We both were: blades can perform very differently for different shavers, and we each were describing our own experience.

The great variation in individual responses to every aspect of shaving means that every traditional wetshaver must willy-nilly be an experimenter: to determine whether a product or technique will work *for him*, he must try it. It may work, it may not, but he has no way to know without trying. Judicious experimentation combined with close observation of outcomes is the most efficient route to learning. The YMMV factor also suggests that the optimal combination for one shaver will probably differ in various ways from another's best set-up—thus the lack of competition. He likes boar brushes, you like badger, I prefer horsehair, and that's that: these choices cannot be sorted into the categories "right" and "wrong".

It follows that if someone recommends a product highly—a razor, a blade, a shaving soap, or whatever—and when you try it, you discover it's awful, you were not tricked or betrayed. You simply came out on the wrong side of YMMV. The guy recommended the product because *for him* it worked great—but that does not mean it will work great for you, though it does suggest that it might be worth a try. Samples—of shaving soaps and creams, aftershaves, and blades—are extremely useful in seeing how the products will work for yourself.

Surprisingly often you'll see a particular product or practice strongly recommended by someone who has not tried any alternative—the recommendation is based on a positive experience with a product or practice but with no experience of any other product/practice. Beware such recommendations and always try alternatives—that is, always experiment.

The idea that someone else's experience is so different from one's own is hard to internalize, especially for those who believe that their own responses are not only "typical" but universal. Yet the idea should be familiar from our experiences with food: we know that a food we love might taste terrible to someone else, and vice versa. Yet even here, some few have trouble believing that their own preferences are not universal—reject fried liver as too awful to touch, and you will at some point encounter a liver-lover who will say, "You just never had it cooked right." No, people do in fact have different preferences, and one must recognize that. I will frequently mention something that works "for me" as a signal that I think it's worth trying but am aware that some others will find that it's not for them. In some cases I can offer an estimate of the breakdown, based on (totally unscientific) polls on shaving forums, but that doesn't help you to know in advance into which group you will fall.

One also frequently encounters a phenomenon I call "YMMV even in the same car": a product that doesn't work for you when you begin shaving may, after six months or a year, turn out to be quite good when you retry it. This is particularly true of blades, as I'll note in that section.

Over time you will work out a custom set-up, procedure, and technique that works best for you. It's nice that it fits you like a glove, not so nice that you have to make the glove yourself. The key is to enjoy the exploration and the experimentation, to delight in discoveries, to develop and test theories, and to increase your knowledge and skill along the way.

It follows that, while almost all men will find DE shaving an enjoyable way to get a fine shave, the YMMV factor means that DE shaving doesn't work for some. For example, some men choose not to shave at all and wear a beard. Some who do shave find that a straight razor works best for them. Starting with a double-edged razor is one standard route to straight-razor shaving: using a DE razor while learning prep techniques and becoming acquainted with the importance of pressure and blade angle, and then moving to a straight razor and developing the skills that straights require (stropping, shaving, and honing), while perhaps continuing to use a DE razor when traveling or for a fast shave when running late. Some like to use a straight razor only the weekends.

Some men, however, cannot use a blade for shaving at all because of skin issues, physical disabilities, or water scarcity. In such situations, an electric razor may be the best solution. (Of course, some men use an electric razor because they don't know that shaving can be enjoyable, so they want to get shaving out of the way while doing something else at the same time—reading the paper, eating breakfast, driving, or whatever.) True to YMMV, though, other men find that using an electric razor is hard on their skin.

The following two sections on straight and electric razors are simply to introduce those alternative: they are not the focus of this book.

Straight razors

Before King Camp Gillette developed the double-edged blade and safety razor, the common shaving tool was the straight razor: a razor-sharp blade with a tang by which to hold it, commonly protected by scales when not in use (though Japanese kamisori straight razors[16] do not use scales).

New straight razors from a manufacturer such as Dovo, Thiers-Issard, Boker, and others are generally not sold in "shave-ready" condition. Almost always it is necessary to send a new straight razor to a honemeister for a professional honing before you can comfortably shave with it. Some dealers (e.g., Straight Razor Designs, Vintage Blades LLC , and Whipped Dog, all listed in the Appendix) offer professional honing on the straight razors they sell so that a straight you get from them will indeed be "shave-ready"—but always ask.

A common introductory route is to buy the "sight unseen" deal from Larry at Whipped Dog: a shave-ready straight with a "poor-man's" strop—novice straight-razor shavers seem inevitably to ruin their first strop in learning how to use it, so this is a good approach for several reasons. The razor will be secondhand and have cosmetic flaws (for example, unattractive scales), but in quality of steel and sharpness of blade, you get a good razor that shaves well: a cost-effective way to test the straight-razor waters. The consensus of skilled straight-razor shavers is that a beginner's best course is to learn with equipment that can be replaced as knowledge and skills improve.

Two useful basic guides to straight-razor shaving are available for free download as PDF files: *The Art of the Straight-Razor Shave*[17], by Chris Moss, and *Straight Razor Shaving*[18], by Larry Andreassen.

Electric razors

As noted above, some men find that an electric razor works best for their situation—for example, because they have rosacea or contact dermatitis or Parkinson's disease or some other condition incompatible with using a blade to shave, or for some reason they must shave without water, or they wish to do something else while shaving.

The common reaction among shavers is that electric razors are something one is forced by circumstances to use. It seldom seems to be a first choice, perhaps because for many men the electric razor is unsatisfactory both in shave result and skin health.

If it's so great, why are cartridges so popular?

Some guys are skeptical because "everyone" uses cartridges. So why was the double-edged blade abandoned? The answer will shock you: money.

In the 1950's Personna (GEM/EverReady etc) invented the Stainless Steel Blade and marketed them for their single edge razors. The blades were sharper but they found that the edge deteriorated quickly and became quite rough to shave with.

Wilkinson Sword was in the forefront with the technology to coat the edge with Platinum, Chromium, PTFE (Teflon), etc., for a smoother shave. Wilkinson held many of the patents and grabbed a considerable proportion of Gillette's market share ever so quickly in the late 50's early 60's — basically, WS blades were noticeably better. And so Gillette made a deal for them to use Wilkinson technology. All of this helped in the demise of the DE as Gillette's patents were coming to an end and they were no longer in the controlling seat. Gillette decided to take a new direction in the early 1960's and cartridge systems would be the end result.[19]

The double-edged blade, now a commodity, is still widely available at low cost, a situation presenting a challenge for companies like Procter & Gamble which must strive to increase profits continually. The solution, as companies see it, is to exploit intellectual-property law[20]. As a result, P&G is working hard in India to offer a single-blade cartridge, the Guard, to drive the double-edged blade out of existence. The Guard is currently quite inexpensive (in contrast to the Fusion 5, for example), but once double-edged blades are gone, price escalation will begin[21]. (In fairness, the safety razors commonly used in India are generally of poor quality and do not shave well.)

The Change Barrier

Resistance to change is common for an obvious reason: change involves risk, and risk means the possibility of failure of one sort or another, whereas continuing the status quo entails no risk of failure: we get what we already have. So our default setting is: "Don't change." But changes do occur, and the interesting book *Changing for Good*[22], by James O. Prochaska, John Norcross, and Carlo

DiClemente, describes their research into why some people succeed in making a big change (for example, quitting smoking). They found that successful change is done in six stages, the first being that one becomes aware that change is possible. By considering how you might change your shave routine you've already begun the process of change: you realize that it's possible, and now you're figuring out the route you'll take. So, although the change barrier is real, the fact that you've gotten this far means you've made it through the toughest part.

Still: recognize that a change in your shave routine is indeed a change, and be patient with yourself through a period of adjustment and learning. The decision to change is generally a conscious decision, but a lot of unconscious work is also required—see *Strangers to Ourselves: Discovering the Adaptive Unconscious*, by Timothy Wilson. Getting all one's internal furniture rearranged, as it were, takes a while. Pay attention to what you're doing and the results of that and you'll quickly pick up the skill—i.e., learn it at the unconscious level.

For some, the transition will go smoothly, and in most cases the novice will see clear signs of progress from shave to shave and from week to week. My own transition went smoothly, though there's a reason I think so highly of My Nik Is Sealed, a liquid styptic I found quite useful when I began but now require about once a month. So if your first few shaves don't go so well as you hoped, remember that you are making a change, that a learning period must be allowed, and focus on the basics: prep, pressure, blade angle, and blade brand, as explained in the following pages. Practice being patient (an extremely useful skill to acquire) and don't expect to gain six months' experience in a week: give yourself time. A good part of shaving is learning not to press too hard, a lesson with general application. Press (down, forward, up, or back, depending on the context) just enough to achieve your goal. A subordinate quickly learns not to press his boss too hard, and a wise boss knows not to press his subordinates too hard. And in learning to shave, don't press yourself too hard—in both senses.

Mindset, an extremely useful book Carol Dweck wrote based on her research, describes well the mindset—the set of attitudes—that best support rapid learning of new knowledge and skills. The book is of general applicability, and if you're interesting in improving your efficiency and effectiveness in learning new things, it's definitely worth reading. The basic idea is that a person who views his capabilities (intelligence, skill, whatever) as fixed and having definite limits will see a failure as a sign he has hit one of those limits; in contrast, a person who views his capabilities as essentially unlimited will view a failure as a sign he's found an area in which he can improve—and the worse the failure, the greater the possible improvement. Indeed, this person views a failure as a source of learning and a direction for improvement. With this mindset, a big failure is *good* because it reveals an area with great growth potential. (If you easily succeed at a task, you have less potential for growth in that area.)

Another aspect of human nature that affects change-tolerance is the difference between "explorers" and "settlers". Explorers look for any excuse to try something new, settlers seek any excuse to stick with what they have. Most of us are a mix: explorers in some areas (physical sports, for example, eager to try any new sport or physical challenge) while being settlers in another (sticking with familiar foods and not wanting to venture beyond meat and two veg).

The settler/explorer distinction is also observed in studies of animal behavior, sometimes called shy/bold[23]. A species benefits from having individuals of both types, the bold to try new foods and new environments, the shy to keep the species going when those experiments turn out disastrously. The different attitudes apparently stem from small differences in brain chemistry, which also turn out to influence one's political outlook[24].

The Fear Barrier

Some have expressed a fear of the safety razor, but it's called a *safety* razor for a reason: the only damage you might encounter are some few nicks while you're learning (in contrast to years of skin irritation and other problems from using multiblade cartridges). With daily practice, your technique quickly improves so that any start-up problems are short-lived.

Indeed, one option is to continue to use your multiblade cartridge razor, just adding to your routine a fragrant lather you create with a shaving brush and a high-quality shaving cream or shaving soap—much more satisfying than squirting some goop from a can of shaving mix. I discuss this approach in the chapter "Recommendation for a Beginner Kit."

Sooner or later, though, you should try a safety razor: a great shave with a blade that can cost less than 2% of what you pay for one Gillette Fusion disposable cartridge.

If you want, you can use a practice blade to perfect your technique before using a real blade: cut a piece of thin, stiff plastic to blade size and use it in your razor to practice using very light pressure and the correct blade angle (shallow, almost parallel to the skin).

In a way, the fear that precedes your first shave with a safety razor resembles the similar fear that precedes your first kiss with someone on whom you have a great crush. Your mind is filled with everything that can go wrong, but you decide to try it anyway, and you get a kiss in return—and suddenly everything is okay. The fears are revealed to be but phantasms, and they vanish in the pleasure of the experience. Don't just take my word for it: give it (shaving) a go. I suggest you take special notice of this fear, because it's like a flower that blooms ever so briefly and only once in your life: after you lather and as you hold the razor before the first downstroke, you may (like many new shavers) feel an odd little thrill of fear, but once you make that downstroke, it's gone forever.

One safety-razor shaver pointed out that, if you were to describe a cartridge razor to someone in the old days, it would sound quite scary: "*Five* blades at a time?! Won't you cut yourself a lot?" Fear of the safety razor can also be merely fear of a new experience, a distaste for feeling awkward when you first begin to learn a new skill.

You also might want to read the following report[25] from someone who's grown accustomed to the safety razor:

Last weekend I went home. My uncertainty about whether to check or carry on was solved by forgetting to pack my Futur [razor] (I was going to decide when I left work whether to leave it in the bag). So my only real shaving option were the things that I had left at home. I wasn't about to drag out the old Norelco, so that meant the Mach 3 that I left there as a spare.

I have not tried a Mach 3 a single time since picking up a DE, so I was actually very curious how it would go. I had often wondered if it was really that much different. After all, unlike some, I remember getting decent shaves with it. But then, I never went against the grain, so my shaves were not that smooth. I did use shaving soap and a brush.

First impression is that this thing does not sit well in the hand. I remembered the metal handle having decent weight, but, well, by comparison [with the Futur] the Mach 3 felt dinky. Also much too light in the head.

With the grain. Ugh. Maybe good soap is not as compatible/does not protect as well when using a cartridge? It felt REALLY scratchy. Not tearing up my face or anything, just not pleasant. Much to my surprise, I realized that even with three blades, the one-pass N-S result was not as good as I can get with many DE combinations. So I decided to keep going, and see if my improved technique and good soap would allow a good multipass shave.

I did three passes, but never fully against the grain because I was getting too much irritation going across. With a Feather DE blade in any decent razor, this would have left me with a near BBS [baby-bottom smooth] shave. With the M3 it was good, but not great. But the real problem was irritation. My skin simply did not look happy. And sure enough, there came the red bumps.

I had to back down to a one pass with the grain the next day, and the third day just did not shave at all.

So, the conclusion is that a DE really does get me a MUCH better result, both in closeness and comfort. What is interesting about this, though, is that this is coming from someone who was perfectly happy with his Mach3 and saw no need to change. I only tried a DE because of the price of stupid cartridges, and the guy love of gadgets.

And, more recently, this note, under the title "What was I thinking?"[26]:

I've just returned from a week in DC. Given that I have a few Mach 3 blades lying around, I decided to take these instead of my DE. Not only that, but I used a can of Nivea shaving foam. It's been some time since I used a combo like this, and my face didn't thank me one little bit!! It's taken a week of using my usual combo (Progress [razor], Trumper [shaving cream], and Rooney [brush]) to calm my face down and get rid of the ingrown hairs. Needless to say, none of the offending items accompanied me on the flight home and all my remaining Mach 3 blades have been sent off to a good home. Don't think I'll make that mistake again…

On a positive note, it has made me appreciate more the whole shaving 'experience'.

The experience of returning to a multiblade cartridge after becoming accustomed to a DE razor seems to be universally disappointing[27].

Beyond the beard

Traditional wetshaving can also be used to remove hair from the body beyond the beard, and it offers advantages over other approaches such as waxing (painful), permanent laser hair removal (costly), or using depilatory creams or lotions (applying to your skin caustic chemicals strong enough to dissolve hair). Many women find shaving with a DE razor works extremely well[28], and many men shave their heads using a DE razor (or a single-edge razor—the GEM razor discussed later uses a single-edged blade, and the correct angle is achieved when the razor's flat head is held directly against the skin—easy to feel even if you can't see the razor, especially helpful to head shavers). Several women have commented that their legs are significantly smoother when shaved with a DE razor than when they used a multiblade cartridge.

Whenever you use shaving to remove hair, the same basic rules apply:
- Use good prep so the hair is easy to cut.
- Make sure you use light pressure with the razor.
- Maintain the correct blade angle.
- Use an aftershave to soothe your skin.

Some differences will be noted. For example, the scalp seems less sensitive than the face, and beard hair is generally stiffer and tougher than hair on the head, so blade selection is less an issue for head shavers than for beard shavers. Head shavers generally have found that a regular double-edged razor works quite well, but some prefer a single-edged razor like the GEM, whose shaving position is easy to maintain by feel.

In shaving the farther reaches of the body—the legs, for example—a long-handled razor can be helpful—though many prefer a long-handled razor even for shaving the face or head. A long-handled Lady Gillette is easily found on eBay with a "favorite search," or you can buy new a Mühle Sophist, Edwin Jagger Chatsworth, or Lord L6, the last being quite inexpensive.

The key is to understand the importance of prep and to use a quality shaving soap or shaving cream and a brush, working up a good lather wherever the shaving is to occur—beard, upper lip, legs, armpits, head, arms, chest, or crotch. The lather makes the hair easier to cut, producing a better shave (and a more pleasant shaving experience) even if you use a multiblade-cartridge razor. Not only do good soaps and creams produce a lather that makes the stubble easy to cut, thus improving the experience, they also come in a wide variety of fragrances that make the entire task more pleasant. (Shave sticks, described later in this book, are a convenient form of shaving soap for the legs.)

Using a DE safety razor in place of a multiblade cartridge razor, the experience becomes (as skill improves) even more pleasant and effective. It's probably best to practice the moves using an unloaded razor (no blade) to get an idea of angle and position. If you make a little fake blade as described above, you can feel the (dull) edge, which helps to judge the angle.

Aftershave care is also important. One woman noted that she liked shaving her legs with a DE safety razor except that afterwards her legs itched. I suggested that she try an aftershave balm, such as Neutrogena Post-Shave balm, and that solved the problem.

FOUR

What to expect

BASED on what many shavers have experienced, you can expect something like the following.

You initially feel skeptical of the idea, but that's followed by the thought that you *really* do not like shaving the way you shave now, and your skin is in terrible shape. So, you think, why not give it a go?

You order a razor, either from an on-line vendor (see Appendix) or on eBay[29] or through the Buy/Sell/Trade section of one of the shaving forums. (You may even get one from some family member.) You go to the drugstore and get a cheap brush and shaving soap. You buy any convenient double-edged blade—because the blade is so cheap, it doesn't seem all that important.

You lather up and—very carefully—pull the razor down your cheek. You try to remember what you've read about the correct angle, and you try to exert very little pressure. (Light pressure is hard to learn for cartridge shavers who have been using firm pressure to try to get a close shave—and to make that expensive cartridge last just a little longer.)

You finish, perhaps with a nick (but maybe not: the first shave is done *very* carefully) and—on the whole—not bad. In fact, it was sort of interesting.

You decide to check in at the shaving forums—to read more and also perhaps to brag a little. So you go to one of the forums listed in the Appendix. You post the results of your experience, and you start reading.

You suddenly realize you've spent more than an hour reading messages in the forum, and you now understand quite a bit more about the process, including some ways to improve your technique.

You order a blade sampler pack so that you have a large number of different brands of blades to try in addition to all the brands you can find locally in the drugstore, and you order a better brush and a shaving cream or soap.

Within a week of your first shave with the DE razor, your shaves are getting progressively better and the nicks have become rare. If you do get a nick, you check pressure and blade angle and resume.

When you encounter a problem or difficulty, you post a question on Wicked_Edge or one of the shaving forums. You usually get advice from someone who had the identical problem and figured out a solution.

You start to really get the hang of it. You've spent some time reading the forum and eyeing the various choices of razors, brushes, soaps, creams, and aftershaves. You've found in the sampler pack a blade that seems to work well for you, and already you can tell that this blade does a better job—or maybe your technique is improving—or both.

You are learning so much, and it's so interesting—fascinating, even— that you eagerly tell your significant other all about it. You observe a certain amount of rolling of the eyes, whatever that means.

Now, as you read the forums, you occasionally find a question from a newbie that you can answer.

One day, after a couple of weeks, you feel your face after shaving and realize that it's smooth—and not just "smooth," but baby-bottom smooth! In every direction! You rub your chin and cheek and feel no sign of whiskers or stubble—you can't even tell when you're rubbing against the grain.

And there's no razor burn! Your face is totally comfortable as well as being totally smooth. All through the morning you surreptitiously feel your face, and you find yourself thinking of tomorrow's shave—which soap or cream to use, which aftershave…

You're hooked[30]. And the learning process continues for quite a while— often taking the form of a gradual awareness. When I first started using horsehair brushes, for example, I thought they were okay, but over time, I began to awaken to their particular virtues, distinct from those of boar or badger brushes, and now I'm quite fond of them. Or when I first got one of the recently designed Edwin Jagger DE razors after using Merkur razors: initially, I barely noticed the difference, but as I continued to use the EJ razor, I gradually became aware that for me the shave was easier and better: the EJ head fit my shaving style better, but at first I didn't realize it. Another example, with J.M. Fraser shaving cream: at first it was just another cream, but over time I began to realize it was curiously effective for my beard, a tad better than most for me.

So take your time and give yourself a chance to find the particular virtues of whatever products you're using. And remember the YMMV principle: another's experience with the product may not match your own. Another person will have a different sort of skin, a beard of a different type, his prep and technique will not be same. Give yourself time to discover your own style and what fits best with it.

FIVE

Where to buy & when to make

AS traditional wetshaving becomes more popular, it becomes a market that attracts large corporations. Procter & Gamble's Art of Shaving stores represent an effort to co-opt the trend, selling wetshaving products but still promoting the most profitable shaving items (the multiblade cartridges). However, in addition to that wolf in sheep's clothing, you can find many excellent on-line vendors that specialize in traditional wetshaving (see Appendix for a list of vendors).

Nowadays many new shavers (especially in the US but also in other countries) turn to Amazon: one-stop shopping and, with Amazon Prime, "free" two-day shipping. But I encourage you to look beyond Amazon, whose offerings are limited in range and sometimes of indifferent quality.

Let me suggest some ways to shop wisely using non-Amazon on-line vendors. First, look for free shipping offers from other vendors. For example, every few months The English Shaving Company (home of the Edwin Jagger line of products, but with many other brands as well) offers free shipping worldwide. Also, many on-line shaving vendors offer free shipping year-round for orders that total more than $25 or some other minimum.

In addition, look closely at prices. Shipping must be paid by someone, and frequently items on Amazon are priced higher than on a site that charges for shipping, the higher price being about the same as the lower price plus the shipping cost—coincidence? This often happens with vendors selling through Amazon as a portal and eager for the "Prime" designation. In such cases "Prime" saves nothing. For example, today Amazon lists Musgo Real Glyce Lime Oil soap, a pre-shave soap I like and will discuss later, for $12/bar with free shipping. BullgooseShaving sells it for $6.50/bar and you pay shipping. If you order two bars (one to use and a spare), using Amazon Prime costs you more.

If you must pay shipping, or if you're trying to order enough to qualify for free shipping, look at adding to the order some consumables that you eventually will need and use up in any event—aftershaves, shaving soaps or creams. Even if you still must pay shipping, by adding a few items to the order you can greatly reduce the shipping cost per item when the increase in shipping is small: every item you add drives down the per-item shipping cost.

Another good way to reduce your shipping cost: Place a single order together with a friend or friends. The shipping fee, split among you, will be small, and moreover the combined order may qualify for free shipping by exceeding the minimum for free shipping. This would be a pain if you order every week, but shaving supply orders tend to be infrequent: every few months, typically. (A tub of soap or bottle of aftershave lasts for months, and a razor lasts a lifetime.)

Also, step back and look at the actual cost of shipping. Consider that a product from an independent vendor (e.g., one of the artisanal soapmakers) may simply be unavailable elsewhere, so if you're going to get it, you have to pay shipping. But how much is the shipping cost compared to, say, a Starbucks special coffee that can easily cost $5? Is getting a special soap or aftershave unavailable on Amazon worth foregoing one or two coffees?—especially since you help an independent vendor who offers special items. I just placed an order with an Irish vendor, and the shipping cost (for a brush and tub of shaving cream) came to $6.04 for airmail delivery to California: perfectly reasonable.

Also look for local retail stores that carry traditional shaving equipment. Procter & Gamble's Art of Shaving stores are appearing in more malls and other locations, but their stock is limited and overpriced (in comparison to other sources), and the staff generally are not knowledgeable about wetshaving.

For shaving hardware—razors, mugs, and brushes—your best bets are independent knife/cutlery stores (the kind with crowded displays) and some pipe/cigar/tobacco stores of the traditional sort. Department stores, particularly high-end department stores, often offer a good range of shaving soaps, shaving creams, aftershaves, and sometimes shaving brushes. Razors are less likely to be found, and the razor selection in such stores is generally quite limited.

Double-edged blades can be found at some drugstores as well as at discount stores like Wal-Mart, but selection is limited and blades are costly, so most shavers buy their blades on-line. Once a shaver knows for sure which brand works best for him, it's wise to lay in a large stock. Stainless, coated blades will last indefinitely if stored in a dry place. (Some shavers buy 100 or so of a brand before they know whether that brand is a good brand for them. That works about as well as you'd expect.)

Occasionally you can find an independent drugstore with a selection of traditional shaving equipment and supplies, and sometimes the selection may be excellent if the drugstore is located in a large city. For example, Pasteur Pharmacy in New York City is good, and Leavitt & Peirce on Harvard Square is exceptional: friendly knowledgeable staff and good stock. Merz Apothecary in

Chicago is another fine store. (Online, it's Smallflower.com.) Take a look around your city, or inquire in the shaving forums to find local stores.

For soap and brushes, check out Bodyshop (they give out free samples if you ask for it), Bath & Bodyworks, Whole Foods, Target, and large drugstores.

Whenever you look for traditional wetshaving equipment and supplies in any brick-and-mortar store, be sure to ask about the items you want. For one thing, they may be stored in a drawer because counter space is valuable and few buy such things. For another, retail-store operators are a desperate lot nowadays, and you can be sure that they will be pay close attention to your request—and if they hear something similar a few times, who knows? You may return to find a display case filled with razors and shaving brushes.

For vintage razors, you can occasionally make a lucky find at flea markets, thrift stores, antique stores, and the like—and, of course, you should ask your relatives about old family razors, used by your grandfathers or your uncles or great-uncles—such requests will often turn up a treasure: a vintage razor in excellent condition that comes with a history and family connection.

Think also about what's outside the frame. Roger Fisher and William Ury, in their excellent and invaluable book *Getting to Yes: Negotiating Agreement Without Giving In*[31], describe how a seller "frames" an offer: the seller learns what the buyer values and includes "in the frame" (i.e., focuses attention on) the benefit the buyer seeks, while putting "outside the frame" compensating charges so the seller still achieves his or her profit goals: in a way, a win-win situation.

For example, if you're buying a car, as soon as you ask about the size of monthly payments, the seller knows that if he minimizes monthly payments, he can readily jack up interest rates, reduce the trade-in offer for your car, and perhaps even cut options. If you focus only on monthly payments, you will accept a deal that costs you more than if you had looked at the total package.

Amazon does this by having you focus your attention on "free shipping." As noted above, quite often the "free shipping" is accompanied by a higher price. And you point out to a friend an independent vendor's lower price, the response often is, "Yeah, but then you have to pay shipping," without even figuring the total amount or considering how to minimize shipping costs. Because the offer is framed with "free shipping," many neglect to look at the full picture. Indeed, you might fail to notice that the range of products available on Amazon is *much* less than the range available from independent vendors, and many wonderful specialty items are not offered on Amazon at all.

The entire field of behavioral economics draws heavily on discoveries by Daniel Kahneman and Amos Tversky on how people *actually* make decisions (which turns out to be very different from the rational maximizers that economists were using as a basis for their theories). Dan Arley, in his intriguing book *Predictably Irrational: The Hidden Forces That Shape Our Decisions*[32], offers a wonderful example: the use of a decoy choices. The book itself is worth reading (if only to become aware of how your choice is manipulated by cunning marketers), but take just one example:

The Economist offered three subscription options:

a. Internet-only subscription for $59

b. Print-only subscription for $125

c. Print and Internet subscription both for $125

Pretty easy choice, eh? His MBA students at MIT's Sloan School of Management chose as follows: option a: 16; option b: 0; option c: 84. Notice that no one chose option b, so Arley dropped that option and offered just two choices:

a. Internet-only subscription for $59

b. Print and Internet subscription both for $125

This time, the distribution was different: option a: 68 (up from 16 previously); option b: 32 (down from 84). Weird, eh? Arley explains in the book why this happens, how decoy choices (such as, "print-only for $125") work, and how this technique is often used to make people choose as the seller wants. It's a book that repays reading.

For the do-it-yourselfer

One option is to make rather than buy, and quite a few shavers enjoy making their own equipment and supplies. Silvertip knots, for example, are available from various sources, and it's not difficult for those with a lathe to turn a nice handle and then use a dab of 3M™ Marine Adhesive to glue the knot in place: a shaving brush you made yourself. (You can use other glues or epoxies, but marine sealant is totally waterproof.) BadgerBrush.net, Blankety-Blanks, The Golden Nib, Penchetta, and Whipped Dog sell badger knots and handle blanks, and a Google search will find more. Another brush option is to restore an old brush[33], and it's satisfying to use a brush whose handle has a history.

Many new shavers want a stand for their brush and razor (though a stand is certainly unnecessary: shavers with a collection of brushes and razors normally do not bother with stands). Homemade stands can be made of wood or plastic, but coat-hanger wire is a popular choice, and for that a wire-bending tool[34] is handy. Home Depot sells heavy-gauge copper wire, which bends easily (especially with the tool) and has an attractive appearance.

Other possibilities for homemade supplies will be presented in the course of the book.

SIX

Shaving step by step

IN the following chapters I explain in detail the process of shaving, following the sequence of the shave. Each chapter focuses on a single part of the shave or a single tool. Optional steps are indicated. YouTube videos made by Mantic59[35] and by betelgeux[36] are an excellent complement to the information in this book.

Grain of your beard

Before you begin to shave, determine the grain of your beard: the direction of its growth. You must know grain direction because your first pass is to shave *with* the grain, your second pass *across* the grain, and later, once you're comfortable using the razor, a final pass *against* the grain (except in areas in which you tend to get in-grown whiskers). You'll probably find that your beard's grain has different directions on different parts of your face and neck. Part of learning to shave is learning the lineaments of your own face.

When you shave with a single blade (rather than a multiblade cartridge), you make 2, 3, or even 4 passes—though when you begin, stick with doing just 2 passes. Multiple passes are made to get a close shave while using minimal pressure: instead of trying to achieve a close shave by pressing hard on one pass, you make multiple passes using light pressure. Too much pressure causes nicks, cuts, and razor burn (scraping away the top layer of your skin). In shaving with a safety razor and a good blade, the weight of the razor is generally as much pressure as you need.

To determine the direction of your beard's grain, wait 12-24 hours after you've shaved, then rub your fingertips (or the edge of a credit card or a cotton ball) over your beard. The roughest direction is against the grain at that point.

For most men, the beard grows downward on the cheeks, so that part of the beard feels roughest if you're rubbing upward. But your beard may have anomalies. For example, I discovered that at the corner of my right jaw, my beard grows horizontally toward my chin: at that point, against the grain is horizontally toward my ear. And at the right side of my mouth, the grain tilts.

The grain on your neck probably has some odd directions. It's not unusual, for example, for the beard on the neck to grow upward, so that shaving downward is against the grain. One reason the neck is so often a shaving challenge is the irregularity of the grain of the beard there. Other reasons are that the razor position can feel awkward and that the skin on the neck is sometimes softer and more flexible and thus harder to shave—stretching the skin by (for example) jutting your chin out will help. Irregular grain is why good prep is particularly important on the neck.

For really gnarly patterns of growth (usually on the neck, but they can occur elsewhere)—especially when the beard grows in whorls, where at least some against-the-grain shaving occurs even on the first pass—the best approach is excellent prep (washing the beard, a hot, moist towel laid over lather or Coral Skin Food: the works). Also, a Slant Bar razor, discussed later, can be an enormous help, especially on the neck: it's not unusual with irregular neck grain for a shaver to experience some irritation, and to some extent this seems due to the way a typical razor pushes directly against the stubble, which irritates the skin. The Slant's easy cutting action seems to slice through the stubble before it can resist. With a regular razor, a useful technique is the J-hook that Mantic59 demonstrates in his video on Advanced Shaving Techniques[37].

Before your first shave, make a small sketch of your face and indicate the grain directions with arrows as a memory aid. Soon, though, you will know the grain of your beard by heart. You can use an interactive diagram[38] to prepare a printable map of your beard's grain.

The winter bathroom

In colder climes the bathroom mirror may show a tendency to fog up in the winter. You can prevent this by applying lather to the mirror, then wiping it off with a towel. Or use liquid hand soap: apply a little to a paper towel and wipe it over the mirror, then use a clean paper towel to wipe until the mirror's clear once more. It will be fog-proof, though ultimately the treatment must be repeated. Commercial compounds like Aquapel Anti-Fog treatment are available, but lather's right at hand and liquid hand soap is cheap.

Another wintertime problem in very cold climates is dry air: cold air doesn't hold much water, and when cold outside air is heated indoors with central heating, relative humidity plummets. If the problem is serious, vaporizers can help, but if the outside temperature is cold enough, the inside air will still be too dry, which affects the quality of the shave (among other things).

The first effect noticed is that the lather will quickly dry on the face—instead of providing lubrication, the lather seems to grab the razor. To avoid this, try making a wetter lather and/or adding a little water to the brush during the shave and working that into the lather on your beard. You can also experiment with adding a few drops of glycerin to your lather. (You can get glycerin at the cosmetics section of a healthfood store; glycerin from plant sources is readily available if you wish to avoid animal products.)

If you use a shave stick, you may have to dip it in water—the water on your face following the beard wash at the sink (or after simply wetting your beard if you find your shave goes better without a wash) will dry so quickly that the shave stick starts to feel tacky. With relative humidity that low, dipping the shave stick makes sense. With normal humidity, that step is unnecessary since the water on the beard is sufficient to wet the stick.

With extremely dry air, you probably will want to look for shaving products that will help moisturize your skin: shaving soaps with lanolin or shea butter or avocado oil or other moisturizing content, and aftershave balms, discussed in the section on aftershaves.

Skin sensitivities

Many men erroneously believe that they have "sensitive skin" because their skin's health has been damaged by using dry chemical foam instead of lather and by scraping their face with multiblade cartridges applied with pressure. But some men do in fact have sensitive skin, which reddens and/or breaks out easily when exposed to common products, sweat, sunlight, or the like.

If your skin reacts strongly when you use particular products (a soap or an aftershave or the like), the product may include ingredients to which you are allergic to some degree. Some guys, for example, find that their face turns red and hot—even a burning sensation—after using a soap or aftershave that includes (say) sandalwood, or rose, or lime (or other citrus). I don't recommend Proraso's (quite good) menthol and eucalyptus shaving cream because so frequently a guy would report that his skin could not take that combination. In contrast, Taylor of Old Bond Street Avocado shaving cream seems rarely to cause any reaction—in fact, I cannot recall reading any problems with it.

Some artisanal soapmakers use essential oils in sufficient concentration to bother some guys' skin. Two that have been mentioned in this regard are the QED and Scodioli soaps, so for those you might want to request samples for testing. I've never had a problem with either, but: YMMV.

If you know or suspect your skin might truly be sensitive to some ingredients, take advantage of samples as much as you can and use them to test the product. Rather than testing on your face, smear a little inside your forearm—the crease of the elbow joint is a good spot—and wait for half an hour to see the reaction. A sensitivity will usually show itself within minutes. The artisanal soapmakers sell samples and Garry's Sample Shop (see Appendix) offers samples of a wide range of commercial shaving products. Trumper and Taylor of Old Bond Street sell very good sampler kits, well worth the price. To make lather from a soap sample, you can use it like a shave stick, rubbing it on your beard, or hold it in the palm of one hand, brushing briskly to load the brush.

If you already know that you have skin sensitivities—for example, you cannot wear wool against your skin—keep those in mind as you shop for shaving products. A person allergic to wool might find, for example, that animal-hair brushes (badger, boar, and horse) are less pleasing to use than one of the new synthetic "artificial badger" brushes—and fortunately artificial badger brushes are excellent and perform as well as their natural counterparts. He might also find that Mitchell's Wool Fat Soap, a truly excellent shaving soap, is not for him—and at the least should try a sample before using a puck.

I find Musgo Real Glyce Lime Oil soap (MR GLO) a superb pre-shave soap, but some guys have skin that reacts badly with the lime oil. Several reported some burning sensation with MR GLO but found when they less—for example, when they washed their beard with the soap using just their hands rather than a washcloth and/or brush, and using less of the soap—they had no further problem and their shaves were still improved. Again, there are good alternatives, which I'll discuss later, but a person with this sensitivity should test carefully any shaving product using lime, a popular fragrance.

Hard water reacts with soap to form a sticky scum, which can also cause skin problems. I later describe workarounds to avoid soap scum, but keep that issue in mind if your tap water is very hard. Extremely dry air, as noted above, can also affect the skin's health, and using a good moisturizer can help there.

As noted, some products seem more apt to trigger reactions— sandalwood, for example, or lime. Some men have reported that their initial use triggered a reaction, a second use less of a reaction, and by the third or fourth use, their skin no longer reacted at all. Other men see no diminution of the reaction—YMMV in action.

The alum block, a post-shave skin treatment, triggers a skin reaction in a few, though most experience no problems. It also seems effective against acne.

Most shavers do not experience any skin reactions at all—I fall into this lucky (and large) group. Those who do have skin sensitivities learn quickly which type of products to avoid.

In addition to sensitivities, consider insensitivities as well. If you use a cologne daily, your nose in time becomes habituated to the fragrance so that you yourself no longer smell it. Some, though, apply enough so that they can smell it well even when their nose is habituated, resulting in fragrance overload, so that others can smell them from twenty paces away. Be aware of the problem and avoid gradually increasing the amount over time.

Because some are quite sensitive to fragrances—to the point of allergies—it's good to avoid fragrances if you will be cheek-by-jowl with strangers, as in airline travel, elevator travel, and the like. Modesty in fragrances is becoming. When I travel, I use an aftershave having no fragrance or only a short-lived fragrance, like the Thayers witch hazels and aftershave.

Beyond skin sensitivities—which are allergy reactions—the skin can also be damaged in time by some ingredients—menthol, for example, is generally regarded as damaging to the skin. Sometimes the ingredient itself may be harmful, sometimes the ingredient is harmful only in combination with other environmental factors (e.g., direct sunlight: citrus ingredients such bergamot, bitter orange, grapefruit, lemon, lemon verbena, lime, mandarin, neroli, orange, or tangerine can cause photosensitivity[39]). My skin seems robust and moreover I'm an indoorsy sort of guy, but it's worth looking at lists of potentially harmful substances[40] and to favor products whose ingredients do not include those substances or they appear only near the end of the list of ingredients.

Still, I must admit that I frequently ignore these issues, which in some cases seem to affect only some people. Sodium lauryl sulfate (SLS), for example, is a surfactant and foaming agent frequently used in shampoos, toothpastes, and soaps, and also in at least one shaving soap (Fitjar Såpekokeri). My wife is quite sensitive to this and must search for shampoos and toothpastes that do not include it, but it has no effect whatsoever on me so far as I can tell, despite the dire warnings one can find on the Internet. My lack of reaction to SLS seems to be true for many, given its ubiquity in products—and the FDA's willingness to accept it as an ingredient. So the rule I suggest is to exercise reasonable caution and care, recognizing that the meaning of "reasonable" varies a lot from person to person. Do not be *too* cautious and keep in mind that YMMV.

Animal issues

Some shavers—vegan or not—may wish to avoid products *tested on* animals. But first note animal-based *ingredients* in shaving products.

Brushes rather obviously use animal ingredients, as it were. Badgers in China—the source of the hairs used in badger brushes—are vermin and are killed in any event, but still some will wish to find alternatives. Boar brushes use bristles that are a by-product of animal slaughter—as with badgers, the animal will die in any case, if that makes a difference.

Horsehair brushes, however, are a by-product of grooming, and horses are not only unharmed, they benefit from being groomed. Still, if you wish to avoid animal products entirely, synthetic brushes are the way to go, and excellent synthetic brushes (often called "artificial badger") are now available.

Many of the best shaving soaps are tallow-based, but those are easily avoided in favor of plant-based soaps that use palm oils, for example. However, palm plantations are terribly destructive of animal habitat and a case can be made that, overall, tallow-based soaps are more benign environmentally than soaps that use palm oils.

An important point that many do not understand is that "tallow" is now a term of art: it describes a particular profile (fatty acid composition, degree of saturation, melting point, etc.) for a fat that may well be manufactured from plant products[41].

Many soaps are glycerin-based, and the glycerin is generally derived from plant rather than animal sources. You can check with the vendor for individual products if the information is not published.

Testing products on animals has been a common practice in the cosmetics industry, and animal testing is more relevant to products such as aftershaves. Many companies now state that they do no animal testing, and the artisanal soaps, shaving creams, and aftershaves listed later are from artisans who do not test on animals. However, cosmetic manufacturers and soap artisans generally don't say (probably because they don't know) whether their *suppliers* do any animal testing. The fact is that companies in general *really* do not want their products to hurt people, who are prone to hire lawyers and start class action lawsuits. Animals, on the other hand, seldom sue and thus testing on animals, to ensure that products will not harm humans, continues to some degree. One can exercise diligence, but the supply chain is long and global in scope and to learn exactly what happens along the way is difficult and sometimes impossible.

SEVEN

Prep

THE quality of your shave largely depends on how well you prepare your beard for the shave. A dry whisker, according to Gillette, is as tough as a copper wire of the same diameter—but a whisker, unlike a copper wire, can soak up water and become easier to cut. Good prep ensures that your whiskers are ready for the razor and don't resist being cut. Inadequate prep leaves your whiskers tough, so the blade tugs, catches, and skips, giving you an uncomfortable and scraggly shave, complete with nicks and cuts, and a blade that's now dull. In fact, shaving with poor prep and shaving with a dull blade feel exactly the same.

Shaving resembles painting in that you spend a good amount of time preparing the surface before actually picking up the brush (or razor). The actual painting/shaving occurs only toward the end of the process and goes more or less easily (and works more or less well) depending on the quality and thoroughness of your prep as well as on your skill and the quality of your tools.

A thorough prep, however, does not mean using every possible pre-shave product you can find. Just as in shaving you apply to the razor the least pressure that works, and on an adjustable you use the lowest setting that gets a good shave (rather than the highest you can stand), so in prep the ideal is to find the minimal set of products and procedures that produce a superb shave: efficiency is the goal. Some go at their skin with hammer and tongs, as it were—almost as though they have a grudge against their skin.

Their frustration and search for solutions is understandable if they are coming from shaving with cartridges: obtaining a healthy skin is a challenge if you're using a high-count cartridge razor (high count in number of blades in the cartridge and, because of price, in number of shaves demanded from each cartridge). In this scenario the skin suffers horribly, and the shaver uses all sorts of unguents and nostrums in an effort to repair the damage, but since the damage is repeated daily, it's a losing battle. The single-blade razor correctly wielded, however, is much kinder to the skin, and you'll quickly discover that you can get an excellent shave from the smallest possible number of blades: one blade. Similarly, use as few products as you can that produce a good prep.

Start with just brush and shaving soap or shaving cream as your prep. Add a pre-shave soap later, and see whether it improves the shave. (It definitely did for me.) That may well be enough, but experimentation is good. Test each new addition to the routine, as well as testing different shaving soaps and creams. The goal is a great shave using as few products as needed for that.

Step 1: Shower – but this varies by shaver

For a majority of men, it's a good idea to shave after showering: the hot water and steam of the shower give a good start to preparing the beard for the shave. Some men, however, find that showering just before a shave makes their skin sensitive and prone to irritation; if you find that's true for you, shave *before* showering. I did an informal poll and found that about 60% shave immediately before showering and 40% shave without a preceding shower—they shower after shaving or at some other time (for example, the previous evening).

A moisturizing hair conditioner used on your beard in the shower may help and is worth a try. Look for a hair conditioner that claims to soften hair— conditioners come in different types[42]. And *always* test any pre-shave procedure. In this case, do *not* automatically make using a conditioner a standard part of your routine, but first do a test: shave a week using a conditioner, then a week *without*, then another week with. Or if a week's too long, try doing the same test, for two days with, without, and then with again. See whether it makes a difference for *you*. Use only what works for you—and only as much as you need.

If you shower in the evening, consider shaving then as well. For a novice, an evening shave works well: in the evening, unrushed, he can take his time as he masters technique. And since the ritual of wetshaving is relaxing, as noted above, it's a fine prelude to a date night.

Some guys use a facial scrub as part of their routine. If you're switching to DE shaving, ditch the scrub for now: the shave itself is exfoliating, and your skin can profitably do without the additional agitation. If you believe you must use a facial scrub, skip shaving one day a week and use the facial scrub on that day. Too much care can be as hard on the skin as too little.

Step 2: Wash your beard

Even though I've just showered, I still wash my beard at the sink with soap and water before lathering. Some get a better shave if they don't do this step, instead just rinsing their face. You must experiment to find what works best for you. Note that hard water forms a sticky scum from soap, so if your tap water is hard, use distilled water for this step. (See the later section on water.)

The pre-shave soap that I've now used for several years is Musgo Real Glyce Lime Oil soap (which I call MR GLO), specifically designed as a pre-shave soap. The identical soap is available also as Ach. Brito Glyce Lime Glycerin soap[43] at a lower price. (Both Musgo Real and Ach. Brito are owned by Claus Porto; the only difference between the soaps is the label.) I tested these soaps using the "week with, week without, another week with" test, and they passed with flying colors: they noticeably improved the shave. 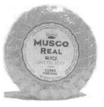 Some don't see it, possibly due to having hard water. Note that MR GLO is **not** a shaving soap and doesn't create a lather: it is a *pre-shave* soap. Use a shaving soap or shaving cream to make lather.

Some find that their skin reacts to the lime (or another ingredient), becoming red and hot. If you think lime may be a problem, try a sample (from Garry's Sample Shop) and test it as noted earlier, in the crease of your elbow joint. If you do have a reaction, try another high-glycerin soap.

I wrote a brief article on several alternative pre-shave soaps[44], all high-glycerin soaps. The glycerin soaps sold by Whole Foods under its 365 brand work particularly well, and those currently cost less than $2/bar and come in a wide range of fragrances. Proraso's Sul Filo Del Rasoio pre-shave soap is, like MR GLO, specifically designated for pre-shave use, and it works well, but less expensive alternatives are also good. Dr. Bronner's soaps, liquid or bar work well; I prefer the bar. One warning on glycerin soaps: they melt easily. In a hot car in the summer, the soap can become more than soft.

Wash your beard with the soap, using your hands, then *partially* rinse with a splash; then apply lather (from a shaving soap/cream) for a fine shave.

Zach (who provided the boar-brush comment later) even uses Dr. Bronner's liquid soap as a shaving soap—either applying it and working up a little lather or simply rubbing some of the liquid soap over his wet beard and starting to shave. He suggests not rinsing after the first pass and not applying more soap: just continue shaving. YMMV.

Some shavers have experimented using a scrubby shaving brush with their pre-shave soap, **not** to work up a lather but to do a better job of scrubbing skin and beard than when just using their hands. Others find the brush too rough and get a skin reaction—for them, simply using their hands works better. You can also try washing your beard using pre-shave soap with a washcloth, but don't scrub hard—and do rinse only partially: the glycerin contributes lubricity.

I recommend against shaving in the shower, but some men prefer that, so if they use a high-glycerin pre-shave soap, it will be used in the shower. However, the soap must **not** be kept in the shower: glycerin is hydrophilic, and a high-glycerin soap will not long survive a high-humidity environment like a steamy shower: the soap will show beads of water on its surface and soon turn to mush. A bar of MR GLO lasts me exactly 3 months, shaving 6 days a week at the sink; kept in the shower, a bar lasts about a fortnight.

Obviously, since you're running a sharp blade over your face, your face should *definitely* be clean. No grime, if you please.

Step 3: Apply a pre-shave [optional]

Before you lather, you can apply a pre-shave to your wet beard. With any of the pre-shaves, be sure to try shaving a week with it, then a week without, then another week with, to see whether it actually helps your shave. Some do find a pre-shave helpful, but others do not. Pre-shaves have never helped my shaves.

Compare the shave that you get when using your pre-shave before lathering for the first pass only and when using it before lathering for each pass: some find their pre-shaves work well only if used before each pass.

Another technique is to apply the pre-shave let it sit—some leave it on as they shower, others apply it and then use the hot-towel treatment (though then it may be that the perceived benefits are from the hot towel, not the pre-shave: experiment.)

I use no pre-shave treatment beyond a pre-shave soap. That and a good lather, allowing time for the lather to work as I brush it into my beard, result in a fine shave for me. I did, however, experiment with all the pre-shave options.

Pre-shave creams/gels

Proraso, an Italian company, makes Proraso Pre- and Post-Shave, a cream that can be used both as a pre-shave and an aftershave. Most apply it only once, before lathering for the first pass, and then leave it on for about five minutes before lathering. Some apply it before showering, and leave it on in the shower. As the name says, it can also be used as an aftershave.

Crema 3P and PREP Classic Cream are Italian pre-shave creams similar to Proraso's. Another Italian pre-shave is a gel: Floïd Sandolor Preshave Gel. Taylor of Old Bond Street (aka TOBS) makes a pre-shave herbal gel that some men with tough beards have found effective. After the beard is washed and rinsed, rub the gel into the wet beard and then let it sit for a minute or two. You could do this step before the shower, for example. Then lather on top of the gel and shave as you normally do.

The Shave Den's pre-shave balm is perhaps more related to a pre-shave oil, though it is a thick paste. The ingredients are shea butter, lanolin, jojoba oil, avocado oil, sweet almond oil, vitamin E, and fragrance (sandalwood and oakmoss). Rub it into your beard before showering and perhaps also apply a hot towel, then lather. Samples are available if you wish to experiment.

Trumper Skin Food

Geo. F. Trumper's Coral Skin Food, available also in Lime or Sandalwood, is normally used as an aftershave balm and skin treatment. Dr. Chris Moss, mentioned earlier, discovered that Coral Skin Food makes a very good every-pass pre-shave, applied to the wet beard just before lathering for each pass. At Trumper's barber shop, Coral Skin Food is applied to the beard and then covered by a hot towel (as described below). Coral seems to work better than Lime or Sandalwood. Note also that a few drops of Skin Food atop puck or brush seems to alleviate lathering problems with some soaps, such as Mitchell's Wool Fat.

100% glycerin

Dr. Moss noticed that Skin Food uses glycerin, so he tried a few drops of glycerin as an every-pass pre-shave. It had much the same effect as Coral Skin Food, but at a much lower price. Healthfood and drug stores carry 100% glycerin[45].

Pre-shave oils

I've never liked oils as a pre-shave (though later I discuss their use as a post-shave oil, for the final polishing pass), so I don't have much to say about them save that they exist. It's not clear to me that they're compatible with a good lather. When I've tried them, I have found that the lather has suffered and the shave was not improved. Your experience may differ—some guys love them—so you may want to experiment with using them.

If you do want to try a pre-shave oil, try using a few drops of jojoba oil or olive oil, recommended by various shavers. Grapeseed oil also gets high praise: it is high in linoleic acid, which is anti-inflammatory, moisturizing, and anti-acne.

Pacific Shaving Company's All-Natural Shaving Oil seems to include some emulsifier so that it doesn't feel so oily as other shaving oils. The fragrance of Nancy Boy Pre-Shave oil is good. Truefitt & Hill make a highly regarded (and expensive) pre-shave oil. The Art of Shaving pre-shave oil is generally disliked as being too gummy, but of course this is shaving: some guys like it a lot.

Pre-shave oil is one of the items for which you can find many recipes on-line[46]. On reddit's Wicked_Edge sub-reddit, indiexsunrise offers one recipe[47], which he has kindly permitted me to quote:

1 part jojoba oil

1 part vitamin E oil

1 part castor oil

2 parts glycerin

1 drop of your favorite essential oil for fragrance

Later in the book I discuss a variety of pre-shave oils that can be used for a final polishing pass, after all lather work is done.

Step 4: Apply hot towel [optional *unless* you get in-growns]

If you get a shave in a good barber shop—and shavers often report that the Trumper shop in London is one of the best—part of the prep by the barber consists of placing moist hot towels over your beard and often your entire face. Sometimes a hot towel is used after applying a layer of lather, or rubbing the beard with Coral Skin Food or with a shaving oil. (Choose one, not all three—well, you could experiment with trying various combinations to see how they work for you.)

The warmth and moisture from the towel helps ready the beard for an easy shave. The basic technique is to wash and lather your beard (or apply Coral Skin Food or a pre-shave oil or other pre-shave preparation), then lay a moist hot towel over your prepared beard (including your neck), lean back, and meditate quietly for 1-3 minutes. The towel's moist heat combined with the lather, Skin Food, or oil softens the beard remarkably[48]. Then remove the towel, apply lather, and shave. You can also tie the towel around your face and neck to hold it in place. If your neck's grain is very irregular, you may want to focus the towel's action on your neck.

If you have a microwave, you can heat the towel by dampening it and putting it into the microwave for 45 seconds. Otherwise, just soak a hand towel under the hot-water tap and wring it "dry." A hand towel is large enough to remain hot for the 2-3 minutes; a washcloth is too small and will cool too quickly.

If you're a true sybarite, spritz a little hydrosol[49] or other fragrance on the damp towel before heating it.

Using a hot towel before shaving is *not* optional if you suffer from razor bumps or in-growns. For those, the treatment is particularly important.

Prep Step 5: Apply lather

THE quality of your lather is a key factor in the quality of your shave. Lather is created from either shaving soap or shaving cream by using a shaving brush and hot water. With experience you can quickly create a good lather, so it makes sense to get a lot of experience in a short time by making test lathers. Be patient and observe carefully the process as you go. The defining characteristics of good lather is that it's dense and heavy with microscopic bubbles. Larger bubbles indicate too much water or water added too fast to be worked into the lather. Your whiskers are easily cut after absorbing water; a thick, heavy lather holds water against the stubble, plus it lubricates the skin so the razor glides easily.

A good lather may be somewhat drier[50] and thicker than you expect—or it may be wetter. Experiment to find the best lather for you. Judicious experimentation is always encouraged—to some extent you teach yourself how to make lather, just as you teach yourself to make free throws: frequent practice and paying close attention to what you're doing and the result you get. Let's look at the components of the process, beginning with the lathering tools.

Lathering tools

Specific tools are used to create lather from shaving cream or soap: a shaving brush, a lathering bowl, and a warming scuttle, the latter two being optional.

Shaving brush

The bristles in a shaving brush are synthetic, horse, boar, or badger—generally bristles of just one type, but brushes are also available that combine horse and boar, horse and badger, and boar and badger. Brushes with synthetic bristles[51] are favored by those with allergies and/or a desire to avoid the use of animal products. Horsehair brushes and boar brushes have been around for centuries and recently are finding new popularity. Badger has long been the standard for expensive shaving brushes, with silvertip badger brushes (the tips of the bristles being white or off-white) as the top of the line.

Some users find that their new animal-hair brush (horse, boar, or badger) has a distinct odor. The odor goes away after brief use, and its departure can be hastened by shampooing the brush (some use dog shampoo) and/or using it with a shaving cream that has its own strong fragrance.

Synthetic-bristle brushes

Synthetic bristles have been significantly improved in recent years. The cheapest brushes still use relatively thick white nylon bristles (like those found in a plastic whiskbroom) and might serve as a brush you keep in your gym locker: they can generate a good lather, but are not particularly well made or comfortable. The best new synthetic bristle brushes are justifiably called "artificial badger." These bristles are thinner than the white nylon, though still resilient, and are treated so that their tips have a fine, soft, bushy finish.

The best of these new synthetic-bristle brushes are completely satisfactory as shaving brushes, with the bristles designed and engineered specifically for the purpose. Moreover, synthetic bristles offer some advantages over natural bristles—men-ü provides a good list of these[52], including drying fast and being hypoallergenic and nonabsorbent.

The five shown in the photo are all good: from left, brushes made by Omega (two brushes: first, the Lucretia Borgia; on its right, model 643147, an excellent first shaving brush), Taylor of Old Bond Street, men-ü, and Mühle. All produce as good a lather as would a badger brush, and all have excellent capacity. After wetting one of these brushes, give it a slight shake so that it will not spill excess water as you begin to build the lather on your beard (the technique I use) or in a bowl.

So far as I can tell, the knots for all the brushes shown (and also for the Edwin Jagger synthetic) are much the same, if not identical, with the differences among the brushes primarily being the handle—except for the Mühle. This Mühle's bristles are somewhat

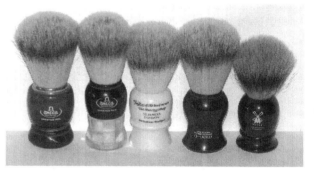

different but they work extremely well—this Mühle (model 39K256) seems to me like a high-quality horsehair brush (which I like). The newest Mühle synthetic brushes, which appeared after publication of the previous edition of this book, are particularly good: a type Mühle calls "silver fibre." The HJM brush made by Mühle is inexpensive and has a soft knot of black synthethic that also does an excellent job. These newest synthetics are particularly nice, but all the "artificial badger" brushes do an excellent job.

Horsehair brushes

Horsehair brushes are enjoying a renascence among traditional wetshavers in the U.S., with a rapidly growing number of fans. Horsehair brushes seem to be favored particularly in Spain and are available in a range of designs, including some made of a mix: horsehair and badger, or white horsehair and boar.

The best source of horsehair brushes I've found is GiftsAndCare.com, listed in the appendix among the vendors. They are located in Spain, and if you do not wish to order from abroad (though I've had no problems at all and shipping charges are modest) some US vendors also sell horsehair brushes.

Vie-Long, a Spanish company, makes a good variety of shaving brushes. Horsehair is finer and softer than boar, slightly stiffer than badger, and as I used them I discovered that horsehair brushes do a particularly good job. Mane hair is softer, tail hair stiffer and more resilient, and the two are mixed in a brush (50/50 and 35 mane/65 tail being the most common). GiftsAndCare will do custom mixes and customs lofts on request: tell them with your order.

Some horsehair brushes have a dyed stripe, and in the first two or three lathers some dye is lost so the lather is slightly grey, but after that all is well.

Even though horsehair brushes fell in popularity around the time of the Great War (because of an anthrax scare[53]), their burgeoning popularity is based on solid performance in the lather department and their modest price compared to badger. Right now, horsehair brushes are my favorites, and they routinely produce exceptionally good lather. It took me several shaves to awaken to this.

In this photo you see an array of Vie-Long brushes. The two on the left are horsehair and badger combined and have a very nice and vigorous action; the remaining brushes are pure horsehair—which, as you see, comes in various colors (as do horses).

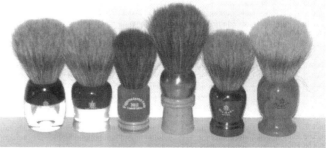

Horses are unharmed in the harvesting of the hair—and indeed it seems grooming is much less traumatic for the horse than shearing is for sheep.

Boar-bristle brushes

Boar brushes have been around since the beginning and continue to be popular. Although the boar brush you find in the local drugstore will probably not amount to much, a well-made boar brush, once broken in, has a pleasant feel and makes a superb lather. Boar brushes are particularly favored by Italian barbers.

Unlike synthetic, horsehair, or badger brushes, boar brushes require a break-in period. The initial week of use makes a big difference for most brushes, but the break-in continues for a long time as the bristles split at the ends, becoming finer and softer. One shaver suggested that you can accelerate the break-in if you use a Suribachi[54] as your lathering bowl. The idea is that the ridges in the bowl help split the bristle ends, making the brush soften and hold more lather. I would *not* use such a bowl with badger or horsehair, though.

Boar bristles, like other natural bristles and unlike synthetic bristles, absorb water (and they absorb much more than badger or horsehair bristles), so you soak them in hot water before use—allowing the boar brush to soak in hot tap water while you shower is the normal practice. Developing a good lather from soap with a boar brush requires a certain amount of practice and rather more vigorous and extended loading than with other brushes.

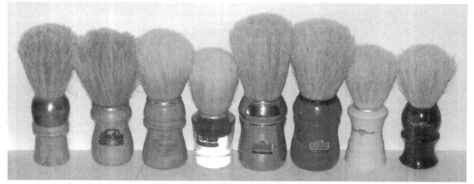

Above is a representative collection of boar brushes—as you can see, I have become fond of boar. From the left, a Vie-Long brush made of boar and white horsehair. This is quite a good brush, though the brass ring around the handle makes a jarring sound when it strikes the side of a porcelain or pottery lathering bowl. The Marvy hard-rubber mug, discussed later, is a good choice for this brush (or similar models that have the same handle).

Next in line are the Semogue 2000[55], the Semogue Owners Club, and another Semogue boar brush, all three being Portuguese brushes from VintageScents.com. Semogue brushes seem to have quality-control problems: I had one Semogue 2000 that worked reasonably well, but the next had a splayed knot that would never close when in use. Based on my experience with them, I recommend against the Semogue brand. I should note that some men do like their Semogue boar brushes—perhaps they were simply lucky in quality of the brushes they got.

Next are two Omega boar brushes: the Omega Pro 48 (Model 10048) and the Omega Pro 49 (10049) to its right are excellent. Some find the Omega Pro 48 somewhat large for face lathering, but the Omega family is large with many options available[56]. The Omega 20107 is somewhat smaller but still a good size with good capacity. Finally, there are two Edwin Jagger boar brushes. For the initial break-in, assuming daily use, count on two weeks for an Omega brush.

The Vulfix Grosvenor is available as a boar/badger combination. This brush didn't work so well for me as the pure boar brushes shown nor so well as the boar-horsehair combination brush. However, the Omega 11047 boar/badger brush is excellent and a favorite of mine (and many others). Soak it for the boar, and it performs like a badger. Its small size makes it a good travel brush and does not affect its (ample) capacity.

Most new shavers will start with a badger, horsehair, or synthetic brush: it's easier to create a good lather at the outset (no break-in required). But boar brush aficionados are enthusiastic, and the price of a boar brush is hard to beat. An enthusiast named Zach wrote a detailed and comprehensive guide to boar brushes[57] that is well worth reading. In discussing this issue with me, he wrote:

> I think that boar is the place to start, especially those new to wet shaving, for a couple of reasons.
>
> One is price over a good silvertip or a synthetic for someone new to something they may not like.
>
> The other is that I find boar is an easier brush to make consistently great lather with, and, that at the end of the day, a good boar brush makes better lather than badger.
>
> And any new thing needs to be learned, so just learn how to use a boar, it won't hurt.
>
> Boar brushes hold less water. Why is this an advantage? Because even boar brushes hold more water than you will need, even boar brushes must be allowed to drain some water or some excess water to be shaken off. Too much water in the mix is the number one problem with bad lather. You're far less likely to have this problem, simply by using a boar-bristle brush. Stated more plainly: if a boar brush can hold too much water for lathering, and a badger brushes can hold WAY too much water, then the ability to hold more water becomes a risk to your lather.
>
> Boar brushes take longer to create a great lather. Why is this an advantage? Because of the simple fact that if you take more time to make lather, you're more able to catch mistakes and compensate for them; also you won't be as likely to miss the 'sweet spot' in your lather. A simple analogy is slow motion; if you can see things happening in slow motion, you can sidestep a potentially big problem. Boar brushes therefore allow for a more

consistent lather than badger does; while this may mean nothing to an expert, novices will appreciate the benefit.

Boar brushes are ideal for face lathering. Why is that? Well, because the lathering on the face part is not all about the face, it's about the hair on your face. Boar works this hair harder, works lather into your pores and into your follicles better, and softens up the hair better by giving it a better workout. Also, contrary to popular belief, a boar brush, when wet, is not prickly, and when broken in, is soft and very easy on even sensitive skin. Boar brushes are somewhat 'adjustable'. Since a boar brush will absorb water, if you let it soak in hot water for 5 minutes while you shower, you will get the softest shave possible with that brush. If you do not, however, you will get a stiffer shave. If you have 2 of the same boar and switch between them every other day, allowing the brushes 48 hours each to become bone dry, they will give you the stiffest shave possible for that brush.

So, in summary:

1) Too much water?

2) Not enough soap?

3) Not enough consistency?

4) Like to face lather?

Answers: 1) boar, 2) boar, 3) boar, 4) boar

Be warned, though, that some boar brushes never work well, so don't assume that problems you may encounter with a boar brush are necessarily your fault. If you do start with a boar brush, try an Omega.

When I first began using boar brushes, I got the impression that they lacked good capacity for lather, as compared to the alternatives. I have since learned—been taught, in fact—that proper loading of a boar brush (brushing the soap vigorously for 30 seconds or more) shows that a good boar brush (the Omega 48 or 49, for example) has ample capacity.

Badger-bristle brushes

Most shavers will sooner or later acquire a brush made from bristles taken from the Asian badger, and these bristles are available in several grades[58].

Badger brushes are made by hand[59]. There are clear differences[60] between pure, best, and silvertip badger brushes, though the meaning of the categories vary by manufacturer. Here are photos of three badger brushes: from left to right: an Omega "pure badger," a Simpson "best badger," and a Rooney "finest badger." Badger brushes with the lighter-

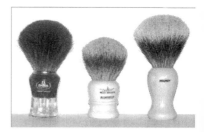

colored tips are softer (and more expensive). The collection of bristles is called the "knot," and the length of the knot is the "loft."

Besides the type of bristle, you should also consider the overall shape of the brush. English shaving brushes tend toward a fan shape, with a more or less flattish top (though slightly domed), but German brushes (the Shavemac, for example) and French brushes (Plisson) often use a domed or light-bulb shape. As with everything in shaving, preferences vary. I like the fan shape but lately have come to enjoy the (domed) H.L. Thäter brushes. From L to R: a domed Edwin Jagger brush, a domed Plisson HMW 12 brush, a fan-shaped Rooney Style 3 Size 1, and a fan-shaped Sabini brush.

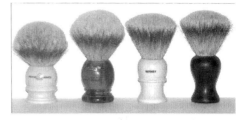

To the right are four German brushes, showing the dome shape Germans seem to prefer: from the left, two H. L. Thäter brushes, a Mühle, and a Shavemac. These are all excellent brushes, though I find the Shavemac too large for my taste.

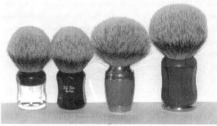

Another difference among brush: the knot may be very tightly packed, or its bristles might be more loosely packed. I find that a tightly packed brush with a short loft just doesn't work for me: such a brush is very scrubby and holds less lather than a looser brush with more loft. A slightly looser, long-loft brush is "fluffy": it's softer, and it holds much more lather. You can, however, quickly make good lather with either type if you load the brush properly (and if the water is soft enough: see the later section on hard water).

The large, flat-topped badger brush at the right is from Enchanté in Austin TX and is designed for Method Shaving (described later). Next to it are three small badger brushes: the Omega 11047 badger/boar brush, an Omega badger, and the Simpson Wee Scot. The small brushes have ample lather capacity for a shave despite their small size, and they make good travel brushes.

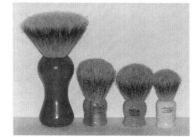

Vulfix badger brushes[61] are popular. I'll compare two brushes from the line to indicate what you look at in brushes other than the shape and material of the knot: the Vulfix 2235 and the 2234. The 2235's longer loft (50mm vs 47mm for the 2234) means that it's a bit more flexible. The 2235 also has a larger knot (measured by the diameter at the base of the bristles)—23mm vs 22mm for the 2234—so it holds a bit more water/lather. The brushes are very close overall. For face lathering the 20mm-22mm seems about right, but of course preferences vary.

Simpson brushes[62] have been a step up from the Vulfix brand, though Simpson has now been purchased by Vulfix. My Simpson Emperor 3 in Super Badger, from a few years ago, is better than my Vulfix. The Emperor's bristles seem to have just the right "give" and density, and I liked its size. Although I still like the Emperor 3 (the largest), as I became more experienced and started building the lather on my face, I got and enjoy the smaller Emperor 2 (pictured). Both are excellent. I have no personal experience with the current Simpsons, but those who have tried them say they are quite good.

Simpson's Wee Scott, pictured above, is surprisingly good. Though diminutive in size, it performs as well as (if not better than) a brush of larger dimension. It holds an amazing amount of lather—HeyRememberThatTime referred to it as "the Tardis of Lather." I found that when it was fully loaded, I had enough lather for six or seven passes (not that I've ever used so many—a three-pass shave works for me—but I kept applying lather and rinsing it off until the brush was empty). The Wee Scot is made of the very finest badger bristles, tightly packed, so the number of bristles in a Wee Scot exceeds that of most brushes made with regular bristles, and this enormous wettable surface no doubt accounts for its surprising capacity. The small size is obviously a benefit when hiking or traveling, but it's also a benefit at home because it offers unparalleled precision in lather placement: a shaver using the Wee Scot no longer risks filling his nostrils when lathering his upper lip. The Simpson Case is the Wee Scot's big brother. I wondered why only the Wee Scot bears Simpson's signature, and Gary Young, of the Simpson family, answered[63]:

> I am lucky to have the honour of having Alex Simpson as my Great Uncle so I can answer this quite easily.
>
> The Wee Scot was the brush that Uncle Alex believed optimised a Simpson brush. Yes, it bears all the hallmarks of a Simpson brush. The Wee Scot was the final part of the apprenticeship. This was the hardest brush to make by hand because of its diminutive proportions. You really had to be confident in all aspects of brushmaking, from turning the handle to forming the knot, to be able to put the Wee Scot together. All of us who were taught

to make Simpson brushes had to make one and have it scrutinised before being allowed to run riot with all the other brushes in the range. Funnily enough it wasn't the current Wee Scot (actually the Wee Scot 2) which we had to make - it was its smaller brother the Wee Scot 1.

This is why Uncle Alex signed the brush because in his eyes, and in ours, the Wee Scot was THE brush that could be held and inspected in chemists, barbers and shops around the world and the holder could see the craft that was used in its making. It was the perfect 'model brush'.

A line of artisanal shaving brushes, some of exceptional beauty, are made by Rod Neep and shown on his Web site Pens of the Forest[64]. I have three and have also given one to my son and to each of my grandsons, with a coin of their birth year embedded in the base of the handle, a nice option that Neep offers. Neep also offers artisanal and custom razors.

The badger brushes made by Rooney[65] are excellent. I first got the Rooney Style 3 Large Super Silvertip, but as I found a smaller brush more to my taste, I got both a Style 3 Small Super Silvertip and a Style 2 Super Silvertip. (Style 2 comes only in Small.) Those are now among my favorite brushes—though, obviously, this can change. This photo from Vintage Blades LLC shows, from left to right, Styles 1, 2, and 3, all in Small. Styles 2 and 3 have a slightly larger handle than Style 1, one reason I prefer them.

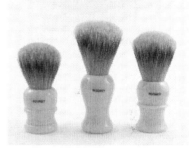

The Style 3 Small has a slightly shorter loft than the Style 2, so it is slightly more resilient. I got a Style 2 Finest and it is today a favorite badger brush—beautiful and functional. (I don't use it in highly pigmented shaving creams—for example, Geo. F. Trumper Rose, D.H. Harris Lavender—since I fear that might stain the pure white bristle tips.)

Rooney also offers the Heritage line of high-quality brushes, and on using an Emilion and a Victorian, I noticed that they, like my H.L. Thäter brushes, showed the phenomenon of "hooked tips" and posted a query (with photos) in the forum ShaveNook.com[66]. Badger brushes with slightly hooked tips present a "spiky" appearance when the brush dries. Brushing the dry brush across your hand restores the usual look, and in use the only difference is that the brush feels extra soft on the face, and if you gently rub the wet tips with your finger, the brush feels "tacky."

At first I shied away from hooked tips, but now I consider them an indication of a very good brush. Gary Young, quoted earlier, notes[67] in the same Shave Nook thread:

'Hooked' filaments can be created way back at the sterilising stage of the hair's 'life'. If the hair has naturally very fine tapered filaments sterilising can cause slight splitting of the hair. Until the hair is used to form a knot and then used by the shaver in the completed brush the 'hooking' doesn't occur. We used to find that some batches of the finer super hair reacted this way, it was something that did create a different feel to the brush - not a bad feel, just a different feel than normal.

That Shave Nook thread includes several close-ups of hooked-tip badger brushes from forum members—Andrew posts some excellent photos[68].

Simpson brushes (measurements here[69]), Rooney brushes, and Omega brushes[70] (measurements here[71]) are all excellent. Both Rooney and Omega Silvertip brushes are amazingly soft and thick—quite a luxurious feel.

Savile Row brushes (from QED) are also nice— soft, not stiff. G.B. Kent brushes[72] are quite nice and soft and do an excellent job building a lather from shaving soap. The BK4, pictured with its box, is the best all-round size. One shaver commented that the BK4 can work up a good lather from a pot roast. ☺ If you like a larger brush, the BK8 would be a good choice. You can also obtain these brushes with black handles. The presentation in the red cylindrical box makes this a nice gift brush.

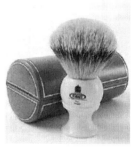

Another line of high-end brushes are those made by Plisson, a French manufacturer who provides handles made of horn, ebony, briarwood, rosewood, and other natural sources, as well as handles of brass and acrylic. Some consider the Plisson High Mountain White the best of all badger brushes. I have one and still like the Rooney 2 Finest better, but this is in YMMV territory.

Morris & Forndran is a British line of shaving brushes that Bruce Everiss mentions with approval[73]. When I used my Morris & Forndran "Blonde Badger," my immediate impression that this is the brush the Simpson Stubby wished it could be. Morris & Forndran brushes are quite high-quality, comparable to Simpson and Rooney brushes.

For a first badger brush, your best bet and the biggest bang for the buck is a Whipped Dog silvertip brush with your choice of resin handle. It's of unprepossessing appearance, but it's highly serviceable and does an excellent job. Like most new brushes, it will shed some bristles in the first few uses, perhaps a few more than a very expensive brush, but bristle loss quickly stops. (If it does not stop within a week, seek a replacement.) I find 20mm or 22mm best for face lathering and a good size with which to begin; experience will show you how the size suits you. I highly recommend the Whipped Dog brushes.

The Frank Shaving brush, typically found at Ian Tang's Shaving Workshop on eBay but also from some vendors, is a good badger brush at moderate prices. Another source of inexpensive but serviceable brushes is Lijun Brushes, again sold via eBay. New Forest Brushes, reviewed by Bruce Everiss[74], are artisanal shaving brushes of traditional design.

Tweezerman is a popular brush on Amazon, but it is of indifferent quality and too frequently the knot falls out after some use. I would not recommend getting that brush. Escali is another brush of borderline quality.

With brush handles made of natural substances such as wood or horn, you should be careful to avoid possible water damage, though in general such brushes do just fine[75]—many boats and paddles, after all, are made of wood.

You may also be interested in the various innovations among shaving brushes[76]—Shavemac, for example, at one time offered a variable-loft brush to allow the bristles to be retracted or extended. It may yet return.

You can even make your own badger brush with supplies from vendors mentioned earlier: BadgerBrush.net, Blankety-Blanks, The Golden Nib, Penchetta, and Whipped Dog. A search on the Web will turn up other suppliers. Look for "badger knots".

Soap brush vs. Shaving-cream brush

Lather is produced from a shaving cream or shaving soap (as discussed below), and sometimes the question arises, "Which brushes are best for shaving cream, and which are best for soap?" In fact, any brush can do a fine job with both soaps and creams provided that the water is adequately soft. You learn how to use the brush to create lather (described later in this chapter), and that's it.

So the distinction between "soap brushes" and "shaving cream brushes" is a red herring. Just pick a brush that *you* like. For me, that's a softer brush with a good loft; for others, it's a stiffer brush with a short loft. One video[77] shows a soft brush quickly working up an excellent lather from a hard soap.

You will notice in the video that he takes his time in loading the brush with soap—the first step of the process, brushing the wet brush briskly and firmly over the surface of the soap to fill the bristles with enough soap for a good lather. Indeed, I would have continued loading the brush for about twice as long as he did. I would also note that his Moss Scuttle was intended to serve as a warming bowl rather than a lathering bowl: as I discuss later, a warming bowl should be small enough so that the brush fits snugly and thus stays warm between passes, so a proper fit means a warming bowl is too small for lathering.

Loading the brush is a crucial step that I discuss later in this chapter. For soaps in a mug or tub (as opposed to a soap in stick form: a shave stick), loading requires a bit of practice to perfect. The usual error is to spend too little time and/or too little pressure when brushing the soap to fully load the brush.

Travel brushes

A travel brush typically allows the user to unscrew the knot (the bristles) and then store it inside the hollow brush handle, thus protecting it during travel.

The Simpson Major Super Badger Travel Brush was my first, and I liked it—a good brush on par with the Simpson's Emperor. (If you do a lot of travel, Em's Shave Place has some nice accessories[78].) Although the Simpson Major's knot looks small, it holds plenty of lather for 4 passes.

Pils, a German company, offers a travel brush, the 503, that has a stainless-steel handle and a silvertip badger knot. It has a "high-precision" feel.

The best travel brush design (in my opinion) is the Mühle travel brush[79]. It's compact and its design expedites drying by putting a large hole just above the stored knot. You can get this brush in nickel-plated brass, quite handsome, or in aluminum in various colors. Aluminum is lightweight but it's also relatively soft, so you must be careful with the threads in those brushes. The knot is pure badger or Mühle's synthetic silvertip fibre, a good idea for travel.

Another form of travel brush is a brush of diminutive size that will fit inside (for example) a plastic prescription pill bottle. The most well-known in this line is the Wee Scot; its big brother, the Simpson Case, is quite good as well. (Em's Shave Place in fact sells the Case with the option of a matching travel tube.)

The Omega 11047 badger/boar combination brush works quite well as a travel brush, and Omega also makes a small badger brush and a couple of small boar brushes (the 50068 and the slightly larger 40033). Despite their size, all of these brushes have ample capacity, and I regularly enjoy using them at home. I recommend that you give them a try. They are not expensive: the two Omega boar brushes run around $6-$7, for example, and the Omega badger/boar brush is less than $20.

My favorite brushes

Each shaver will have his own preferences with regard to every aspect of shaving: methods, equipment, and supplies. Still, I do get asked which brushes I prefer, so here are some favorites. Of the four types, I currently prefer horsehair.

The badger brushes I most often use are my Rooney Size 2, the Wee Scot, the Rooney Victorian, the G.B. Kent BK4, and a Whipped Dog silvertip.

I have a number of other favorites. There's the scrubby crowd: the Simpson Duke 3 Best and two Morris & Frondran "Blonde Badger" brushes.

The Plisson brass-handled size 12 Chinese Grey has an interesting coarse feel and does a fine job, as does the Plisson size 12 High Mountain White. And I like the Thäter brushes a lot.

I'm becoming increasingly fond of boar brushes, particularly those made by Omega: the Pro 48 and Pro 49, the 20107, and the 40033.

I've had excellent luck with horsehair brushes, and I have a collection now that I enjoy using frequently. The horsehair plus badger combination brushes that Vie-Long makes are also good. I find that horsehair brushes perform extremely well. The synthetic bristle "artificial badger" brushes are all excellent and I use them regularly—to me, they are as good as badger bristle.

Care of your brush

If you soak your brush prior to shaving, use hot water from the tap, *not* boiling-hot water. Boiling-hot water will ruin the bristles. I don't soak a badger or horsehair brush—I simply hold it under the hot-water tap until it's full of water—but I do let a boar brush soak while I shower: boar bristles soak up a lot of water and soften considerably. However, in this as in all things, experiment: try soaking your badger or horsehair and compare how it performs when soaked and how it performs if you simply wet it under the tap before lathering.

Lather from shaving cream is slightly acidic. This is no problem during the shave: the lather's water dilutes the acid's action, and the lather's rinsed out at the end. But some, thinking not to "waste" the lather, let it dry in the brush, and the acidity becomes concentrated as the water evaporates. This will over time destroy your brush. Thus it is vital to clean the brush before putting it away. When you complete your shave, rinse all the lather out of your brush with warm or hot water, and then do a final rinse of the clean brush using cold water. (The hot water should not be so hot that you cannot keep your hands in the stream.)

The reason for the cold-water rinse is that the hair shaft is covered with cuticle—overlapping scales somewhat like roofing shingles[80]. In hot water, these scales stand out from the hair shaft; in cold water, the scales hug the shaft tightly. This is one reason shaving with hot water is more comfortable than shaving with cold: hot water opens the cuticle and the whisker absorbs water more readily. And this is why beauticians do a final shampoo rinse with cool water: so the cuticle lies flat and the hair will look shiny instead of dull.

You may want a stand for the brush, but since most stands grip the brush at the base of the bristles (bristles downward), stands can damage the knot. It's better if the stand holds the brush by a groove around the handle, as in some of the Mühle brushes. Simpson states that their brushes should simply stand on the base of the handle to dry after you've rinsed the bristles and shaken it well to remove excess water—no stand needed. (Some also dry the brush on a towel, but I don't bother.) Indeed, if you collect brushes, you would have to improvise a large rack. I use a couple of wall-mounted 4-tier spice racks to hold my collection of brushes (and razors), with the brushes standing on their bases. (In looking at the orientation of the logo on almost all brush handles, it does seem that the makers expect the brush to stand on the base of the handle.)

Over time brushes may become slightly waterproof from hard-water deposits. One symptom is that the lather doesn't seem quite so nice or abundant as previously. Brushes can be easily restored by washing them with a good shampoo and conditioner. Be very careful about the shampoo: some include silicone-based additives that can make the brush less functional. The bad additives generally end in "–cone"; here's a partial list of what to avoid: cyclomethicone, cyclopentasiloxane, dimethicone, dimethinconal.

Johnson Baby Shampoo (very gentle and with a neutral pH) is a good choice—or, instead of using shampoo, soak the brush for 10-15 minutes in warm water to which you've added a splash of white vinegar. The vinegar dissolves the hard-water (calcium) deposits, leaving the bristles no longer coated. After soaking, rinse the brush well, first in warm water, then in cold. Make sure you've rinsed away all traces of the vinegar. Bleach is a *very* bad idea: don't use it at all.

Emily from Em's Shave Place has various reference articles at ShaveInfo.com, including some videos on a brush cleaning method[81] that produces excellent results. You first soak the brush for about 5 minutes in warm (not hot) water with some dishwashing detergent (not the kind you put in a dishwasher, but the kind used in hand-washing dishes), swirling it from time to time. Then mix 9 parts water, 1 part white vinegar and a dash of 100% glycerin (available at a drugstore or health-food store) and soak the brush in that for about 10 minutes. Rinse the brush, and it will now be soft and water-absorbent.

As described in the later section on "Cleaning your razor," you can also use an ultrasonic cleaner to clean the brush—you immerse *only* the bristles, **not** the base of the knot. Gold Dachs makes a shaving brush cleaner[82] that's reported to work quite well. MAC brush cleaner[83] is intended for cleaning make-up brushes, but those who have cleaned their shaving brushes with it found that it did an excellent job.

Cleaning the brush may not be needed if you have soft water and are careful about rinsing the brush after use. And it certainly isn't needed so often as cleaning your razor. Remember that badger, boar, and horsehair brushes are made from actual hair, so don't do things to them that you wouldn't do to your own hair. Synthetic bristles are more forgiving and robust.

Lathering bowl [optional]

I do not use a lathering bowl. I found that for me it works much better to load the brush and then work the lather up on my beard ("face-lathering"). But many shavers like to use a lathering bowl, so I will describe the process here.

Building the lather in a bowl does help you observe the lather as you experiment, trying different proportions of water and shaving cream or soap until you learn to get a lather you like. (I have a strong impression that a lathering bowl is more frequently used with a shaving cream than with a shaving soap.) You can rub the lather between thumb and finger to see how protective and slick it is. Thus the lathering bowl is useful for making practice lathers to gain experience. For example, put a lump of shaving cream about the size of an almond in the lathering bowl, wet the brush and shake it out, then begin brushing the cream.

Because you shook out the brush, the lather will not really form, so add a tiny amount of water, work that in, and check the lather. Continue adding a tiny amount of water, working it well into the brush and lather, testing it, and repeating the process until the lather is obviously too wet. Along the way you will have seen lather at every stage of development, from too dry to just right to too wet. If you do that a few times, you will start to recognize the stage of lather that you most prefer. You can do the same experiment on your beard, but it's easier to observe in the bowl. Once you know the stage you want, you can develop a good lather on your beard or in the bowl.

Because a bowl is normally used as a container, the natural tendency is to think that the lathering bowl's purpose is to hold the lather, into which you dip the brush and then apply—much as a paint can holds the paint that the paintbrush applies. Not so: the lather's in the brush, not in the bowl. The bowl merely presents a surface of a convenient shape for building a lather. This fact becomes obvious when you create the lather directly on your beard.

I first did this on a trip, having opened my suitcase to find a broken lathering bowl. I found that I really didn't need the bowl to make good lather: I could work it up on my beard, and the brush then held plenty of lather for multiple passes, and now I greatly prefer "face-lathering" to using a bowl.

It's difficult to see how the lather's doing if the lathering bowl is white, so use a bowl that's a relatively dark color. Other than that, any roughly hemispherical bowl that's about 5" across and 2.5"-3" deep will work fine. Start with a cereal bowl from your kitchen or visit Target, which normally has a good selection of inexpensive cereal bowls in various colors.

The lathering bowl—important point—should be filled with hot water and allowed to sit (while you shower, for example). Few enjoy cold lather. Empty the hot water from the bowl, rinse the brush in hot water, and proceed. Obviously, you can use hot water from the tap to heat the bowl, even if you're going to use distilled water for the lather. Dirty Bird Pottery makes a lathering bowl that is heated as a scuttle (see next section).

With a very large brush, a lathering bowl may work better than building the lather directly on your beard. A 20mm-24mm brush is a reasonable size for face lathering, as you can work it smartly against your beard, but a really large brush may not get enough action merely against the beard. For large brushes, the bowl lets you work up the lather more easily than on your beard, and also allows you to adjust water amounts.

Another important point: badger brushes hold a lot of water, and if you fail to work all that water into the lather at the outset, you'll find that in the second and third pass the water drains into the lather in the brush, making it thin and worthless. So, *especially* with a brush that's both large and stiff, gently "pump" the brush (and this is where a lathering bowl is helpful), combined with the usual swirling and stirring motions. You pump the brush by working it up and down; this ensures that the water at the base of the brush gets worked into the lather. (I accomplish this now when I'm loading the brush, described below.)

Don't pump the brush so vigorously that you damage the bristles— gently but enough to work the brush's charge of water fully into the lather. Experience will be your guide. Brushes that hold much water will require a bit more shaving cream or shaving soap for a proper lather than a brush holding less water.

Some large-knot brushes, like the Omega Silvertips, are soft and flexible enough so that the pumping action usually happens automatically as you swirl and stir up the lather. With these brushes, no special pumping is required.

Suribachi bowls should be used *only* with boar brushes—and optionally even then: they are not really necessary.

Warming scuttle [optional]

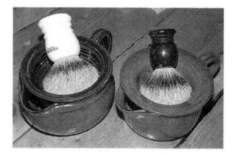

The Moss Scuttle[84] (shown at right) allows you to enjoy warm shaving lather, a real treat. It consists of a brush bowl sitting in and attached to a heating bowl (so it doesn't fall off when you empty the water).

To use: fill both bowls with water as hot as you can get it from the tap. Leave the hot water in the bowls while you shower.

Then empty out all the hot water, and fill only the heating (bottom) bowl with hot water: this will keep the brush bowl hot. Rinse the brush with hot water, then load it with soap or cream and build the lather. After the first lathering, place the brush in the warmed brush bowl while you shave. Then, when you relather before the next pass, the brush and lather will still be warm.

The brush bowl should be too small to use as a lathering bowl—you want the lathered brush to fit snugly in the bowl to keep warm. The Moss scuttle comes in two sizes—small and large (see photo)—and the small size is right for all but quite large brushes. Dr. Moss kindly provides this step-by-step procedure:

My experience is that if you make the water in the scuttle too hot it will encourage the lather to break down. The other thing is whether you are getting the proportions right when you make the lather. Here's the way I use the scuttle:

1. Fill scuttle with hot water in both compartments.
2. Soak brush in the hot water in the inner bowl.
3. Do other stuff - for me this means wash face and strop razor, but for you might include reading New York Post, write angry letter to editor, kick cat, and so on.
4. Empty scuttle.
5. Refill outer part only with hot water.
6. Shake out brush.
7. Place exactly one British Standard Fingertipful of cream on brush.
8. Work brush into inner bowl of scuttle, adding a few drips of hot water as necessary.
9. Make lather on face, dipping brush tip in hot sink water judiciously if necessary (it usually is).
10. Place brush back in scuttle and push down to maximise brush to scuttle contact area.
11. Shave, or something like it.
12. Relather with hot lather. Place brush back in scuttle *q.v. step #10*
13. Shave again in some other direction.
14. Relather for the bits that need it. Place brush you know where.
15. Shave in another direction, removing tiniest traces of beard.
16. Rinse face, brush, and scuttle in desired order.
17. Kick cat.
18. Go to work, pretend to enjoy it.[85]

Georgetown Pottery[86] makes a scuttle that serves the same function as the Moss Scuttle, though with a slightly different design. Robert's Feats of Clay also makes a line of scuttles of good design[87]. Dirty Bird Pottery[88] makes what in effect are heated lathering bowls (and unheated lathering bowls as well), but they also make a "brush holder" that fits the brush snugly enough to keep it (and its lather) warm. The ideal would seem to be to combine the two ideas: a large bowl used for lathering and then filled with hot water once the lather is made, and a smaller brush bowl then placed in the hot water and used to keep the brush (and its lather) warm while you shave. The trick would be to find a mechanism to prevent the small bowl from floating and capsizing.

Dan Straus, a chemist in San Jose, discovered that the Rival Little Dipper makes a fine lathering bowl/brush warmer[89]. It has no heat setting or on/off switch, so he just plugs it in when he awakes, and after breakfast and a shower, it's just right for warm lather.

One shaver has pointed out that a *thick* ceramic bowl will hold quite a bit of heat once it's hot all the way through, and can keep the lather warm for the entire shave. Others put their lathering bowl in a sink filled with hot water. Some find a pair of bowls to use in the manner of the Moss Scuttle. I usually just stand my brush on its base between passes, and the lather stays warm enough for me.

I should add that those who like the scuttle like it a *lot*—for them the warmed lather adds significant pleasure to the shave.

Water

Water is a key component of a good shave, and there's more to consider than you would at first suspect.

Temperature

When talking about "hot" water, it's important to note that water that's *too* hot is not only bad for the brush, it's also a safety hazard. Burns and scalds from hot water are among the most frequent home accidents, and so I've followed the recommendations made a generation ago by then-President Carter: set the hot-water tank's thermostat so that pure hot water coming from the tap is just right for a shower, shave, and dishwashing. This finesses the safety hazard of scalding water, and it saves money: you don't pay to heat water to a temperature too high to use, and then when using it, cool it down by mixing in cold water.

At one time, dishwashers did require extremely hot water from the tap, but nowadays dishwashers themselves heat their water to the scalding temperatures they require. Do yourself a favor and try turning down the hot-water heater to a temperature that allows you to use pure hot water for shaving and shower without discomfort or danger—unless you have a large family and a small hot-water heater. If that's the situation, you may run out of hot water.

If I let the water run until it reaches the maximum, hot water from my tap now runs at 116°F (47°C). I used trial and error, adjusting the hot-water tank thermostat over a period of days until the setting delivered pure hot water at a usable temperature.

Another temperature consideration is whether to shave using hot water or cold water. I consider cold-water shaving a last resort, but in fact some shavers like it, especially in hot weather. They say the cold water tightens the skin and makes the stubble stand erect, thus easier to shave. (Presumably they shave at the sink, not in the shower.) When I tried it, I didn't get as good a lather, and the shave, while okay, did not seem to be an improvement—certainly not enough so that I was willing to abandon the comfort and luxury of a hot-water shave. But experiment: try a cold-water shave some hot day.

Hard v. Soft

Normally you can simply use hot water from the tap to make your lather, but if you live where the water is hard—or if you think the water might be hard—try using distilled or "purified" water, sold cheaply in drugstores for use in steam irons, steamers, vaporizers, and the like. If the lather is then markedly easier to make and more abundant, you have your answer—and a workaround.

One sign that the water is hard is that washing your face with soap leaves it "squeaky clean": the squeakiness comes from soap scum on the skin.

Rather than buying distilled water—it sells for around $1/gallon—you might try collecting and filtering rainwater, or make an air well[90] to harvest dew—obviously something best done by country dwellers. Another nearby source of condensed (and thus in effect distilled and therefore soft) water in many homes is a dehumidifier in a damp basement, but that water may well be contaminated by mold and/or fungus—particularly in a damp basement (which is why the dehumidifier's there to begin with). On the whole, it seems best to buy a gallon of distilled, especially since a gallon can easily last a month.

The best long-term solution for hard water is to install a water softener. Household water softeners generally use ion-exchange, replacing calcium in the water with sodium, so that softened water is unsuitable for drinking or cooking. With these softeners, the kitchen cold water is not softened (or you can mount a reverse-osmosis softener under the kitchen counter to soften water from that tap; this type of softener removes the calcium without adding sodium).

If you do install a water softener, look for one that recycles based on volume of water used rather than on time (every few days). Volume-based regeneration automatically adjusts for periods of low usage (when you're away) and high usage (when you have house guests). Good volume-based softeners use two tanks: while one tank regenerates, soft water continues to be available from the other[91], thus keeping hard water from filling the hot-water tank.

Water with high mineral content is hard on the hot-water tank, the plumbing, and the valves and faucets. It's hard on skin and laundry, leaves deposits (mineral and/or soap scum) on everything (including your skin), and can make the razor blade seem dull: as the water evaporates from the blade, hard water deposits cover the cutting edge. (To prevent this, rinse the razor head in high-proof rubbing alcohol after the shave: the alcohol displaces the water and then evaporates, so there's no mineral build-up along the blade's edge.)

A person using soft water for the first time will often complain that they can't rinse off the soap. What they mean is that when they rinse away the soap, their skin still feels slippery (as wet skin should). What they are missing is the stickiness they felt from soap scum adhering to their skin—that's what they've used as the sign that all the soap (which does make the skin feel slippery) is gone. When using hard water, after rinsing they feel the soap scum that remains, stuck to the skin, and so they don't feel slippery. With soft water their skin still feels slippery, so they believe that must be due to soap remaining. It's not: it's the natural condition of wet skin. (When you're trying to remove a ring that's too tight, you wet the skin to make it more slippery).

If a water softener is infeasible in your situation, you can use the workaround: distilled (or "purified") water heated ahead of time on the stove or in the microwave, or with something like the Sunbeam Hot Shot[92] to heat it in the bathroom. (The Hot Shot brings a pint of water to 180°F in a minute—too hot, so you have to cool it: turn it on before you shower, and by the time you're done it should be about right.) Or you can use a hot-water dispenser like those made by Zojirushi[93]; these maintain water at a pre-set temperature (175°, 195°, or 208° F—all of which are again too hot, requiring cooling). Or the UtiliTEA[94] kettle will quickly heat water to the temperature you set; at its lowest setting it heats water to 125°F. That still requires a little cooling before use, but it presents less of a scalding hazard than the other workarounds.

For a shaver accustomed to hard water a distilled water shave can be astonishingly better[95]. And some who thought their lathers were pretty good are amazed by the difference when they try a distilled-water shave.

Because hard water affects the lather from shaving cream less than that from shaving soap, the idea of a "soap brush" v. "cream brush" probably began with shavers whose tap water was hard. They observed that they got good lather from shaving cream but, *using the very same brush*, they could not get good lather from shaving soap. They then decided that their brush must not be a "shaving soap brush," though the problem was the water, not the brush.

If you are the least bit unsure about the hardness of your tap water (and in particular if you live in a hard-water region[96]—for example, the Midwest or

Southwest of the US, much of Australia (Adelaide's water is notoriously hard), and in the prairie provinces of Canada)—I urge you to try the distilled-water experiment: it's inexpensive and the results might surprise you. And it's easier than it sounds because the volume of water involved is so small.

Using distilled water

Heat about half a cup of distilled water to around 116°F/47°C. You can pour it into a thermos, though that seems overkill: a measuring cup (easy to pour) or bowl of water will stay comfortably warm for a shave. If you use a boar brush, also pour a little water into a cup to soak the brush. You then use water:

- to wash your face with pre-shave soap and rinse with a splash (not a thorough rinse: residual soap contributes lubricity to the lather);
- to make the lather;
- to rinse your face after each pass (two partial rinses and a final thorough rinse for a typical three-pass shave);
- to rinse lather off the razor (pour a little into a cup or bowl for this— for example, use the water left in the cup after soaking the brush).

After very little practice, I found that a good three-pass shave requires only ½ cup water. It helps that only the final rinse must be thorough and that I don't use a moist hot towel (though for that you can use tap water rather than distilled water—and you can also use tap water, even if hard, to rinse off your hands). Using a scuttle can help[97]. Depending on how hard your tap water is, you can try using a distilled/tap water mix to stretch the distilled water, but even if you use straight distilled water, a gallon (at ½ cup per shave) will last for a month easily, especially if you skip shaving one day a week as I do.

In reading the procedure, it might seem bothersome, but with a week's practice it becomes routine: the adaptive unconscious learns and takes over (just as it does for the much more complex tasks involved in getting dressed) so that most of it (using distilled water or getting dressed) is done automatically, with no conscious attention or thought. In getting dressed, for example, you consciously select what to wear, and then the unconscious takes over, putting on the various pieces, tucking, smoothing, fastening, zipping, buckling, tying, and so on, while your conscious mind and attention is on other things entirely.

Minimal-water shaving is also handy when water is scarce, as (for example) on a camping trip. (Surely you shave when camping, right? ☺)

Shower v. Sink

I don't shave in the shower, though a shower shave provides lots of available water: easy to rinse between passes, for example. That's its only virtue, so far as I can see, and that for me is outweighed by many disadvantages. Excess water usage is not a significant disadvantage, assuming that anyone shaving in the shower *must* live in an area with abundant fresh water. Where I live—and in many locations—water restrictions regularly apply and shaving in the shower would be a shocking waste of water. A beginning shaver with a DE safety razor or a straight edge will often take 20 or 25 minutes or more for those first shaves. I shudder to think of the water lost, even with a low-flow showerhead.

Even apart from excess water usage, the shower shave has several significant disadvantages. For one, the noise of the running water keeps the shaver from hearing the auditory feedback from the razor's action, a significant loss. (Of course, some showerheads have a little push-valve to turn water on and off with no change in temperature, so the shave could be done with the water turned off except to rinse—but if you're doing that, why not shave at the sink?) For another, there's no place (at least in my shower) to set out my shaving stuff in an organized way. Brushes should not be stored in the shower, obviously, so for each shave you carry in a brush, then carry it back out. Razors get slippery with soap and are likely at some point to be dropped, and as it falls the blade may cut you—or slice off a piece—and in any event is likely to be damaged, and probably the razor as well. The alum block is water soluble, and high-glycerine soaps turn to mush, so you can't leave either in the shower.

A shower shave probably precludes the cold-water shave, a minor loss. You can buy shower mirrors, though many shower shavers simply shave by feel. If you use a soap mug in the shower, consider the unbreakable Marvy mug made of hard rubber; it's quite a good mug in any case. For a shower shaving cream, Em's Shave Place uses plastic dispenser bottles.

My recommendation: wash in the shower, shave at the sink. But one great thing about shaving: you get to decide for yourself. (I've not read of guys who shave in the tub, though we've seen that in movies—typically in Westerns.)

Running v. Still

When you shave at the sink, shavers typically take one of three approaches:
1. Fill the sink with hot water and use that for the shave: rinse your razor and your beard in the water until you finish the shave.
2. Leave the water running, rinsing your razor in the stream as needed and using that water to rinse your face between passes.
3. Turn the water on as needed to rinse razor or face, then turn it off.

Option 2 is a bad idea, quite apart from losing water you've paid to heat. The shaving problem is that running water makes a lot of noise. Keep the bathroom as quiet as possible when you shave. That supports the contemplative mood, and the silence also allows you to hear the sounds of shaving—the blade cutting through the stubble—which helps you in adjusting blade angle.

I use option 3—my lavatory has a single-lever faucet, so turning water on and off is easy—but some guys prefer the first. Try both to see which works best for you, but keep the bathroom quiet: no fan, no radio, no running water.

Soaking

When you shave, you find yourself soaking various things—your beard, most prominently. It gets soaked in the shower, soaked again at the sink as you wash it, perhaps soaked once more with lather beneath a hot moist towel, and then soaked as the lather is worked in. The more water the beard absorbs, the easier the shave and the longer the blade will last.

Some soak their shaving brush while they shower. Based on my experience, this soaking doesn't seem to help badger, horsehair, or artificial badger, but it's important for boar brushes. Boar bristles absorb a lot more water than the others, and soaking greatly improves their performance. Badger and horsehair brushes become a *little* softer, but for me it's not worth the effort.

Some put a little water atop the puck of shaving soap and allow that to soak while they shower. I tried this, and so far as I could tell, it did not the slightest good. By all means, experiment and draw your own conclusions. (A little Trumper Skin Food or glycerin atop Mitchell's Wool Fat does seem to help.)

Latent lather: Shaving cream and shaving soap

Lather is born from a cream or soap with the addition of water and the action of the brush. Done correctly, the result is far more fragrant and efficacious than dry chemical foam squirted from a pressurized can, and more pleasant than most brushless shaving creams. The traditional method—using brush and soap and cream—does, however, lack cool TV commercials.

The distinction between creams and soaps is not so strict or clear as you might imagine. Soaps come in soft formulations (for example, Vitos Red Label and Valobra are Italian soft soaps, soft enough to mash into a bowl or mug, and produce terrific lather), and some creams—those in tubs—can be quite stiff and soap-like. Figaro, an Italian shaving cream is as firm as soap, and Ginger's Garden shaving-cream soap lathers more like a shaving cream than a shaving soap.

The reformulation problem

Some shaving soaps make a very fine lather: abundant, fragrant, lubricating, protective, and long-lasting. Other shaving soaps are best used as bath soaps: the lather they produce is stingy, non-lubricating, unprotective, and short-lived. The same phenomenon happens with shaving creams, though not to the same degree. Why would any company produce a soap or cream as bad as some you find?

Modern businesses operate under constant pressure to increase profits (example: the multiblade cartridge). So sometimes, due to financial pressures, a soap, shaving cream, or other cosmetic is reformulated to increase profits, thus doing a better job (from the corporate accountant's point of view: a cosmetic's job, for them, is to produce profits—also, some people use them for something). Obviously some reformulations are done in order to improve the product, but surprisingly often a product reformulation's main purpose is to increase profits without sacrificing too much revenue (from customers who stop buying the product after reformulation—hopefully replaced by new customers).

At a marketing seminar, I was told of a large consumer-products company that fell into this sort of trap: their product managers are each put in charge of a product. A new product manager wants to show success, to move up in the organization, and the only measure of success most businesses recognize is that product profits increase. One easy way to accomplish that is to reformulate the product, substituting when possible cheaper ingredients for more costly ones—or just omit the costly ones. (Another strategy frequently used is to reduce the size of the container a small amount, changing the shape to disguise the diminution. Since the container is new, it is labeled "NEW!".)

Careful testing is done after reformulation to make sure that consumers show no significant preference for the old formulation, and once that test is passed, the product is re-released, the profits increase, and the product manager is promoted. In comes a new product manager, eager to make a mark.

The easiest way for the new product manager to increase profits is to reformulate again, using even cheaper ingredients. And so the process continues over several generations of product managers.

Call the original product A, and the first cheaper version B. Customers can't tell the difference. And then there is C, and customers can't distinguish C from B. Or D from C. And so on. But somewhere around F or G, the cumulative difference becomes quite noticeable, with A quite obviously better than G. At around this point product sales fall off a cliff, the product is discontinued, and the last product manager, left holding the bag, is fired or disciplined. But, in general, no actual organizational learning occurs, so the process is continually repeated for other products. (It's extremely difficult to build a learning organization: Chris Argyris devoted his career to figuring out why, producing some wonderful books in the process.)

So this is a general warning: when someone tells you how great some particular cosmetic is, find out when they bought it. In the shaving arena, several soaps and shaving creams have been reformulated over the past few years, not always to the shaver's benefit (though the companies profit from the change). Floris London shaving soaps I bought some years ago are very good, but those who bought their soaps after reformulation have little good to say about it.

It should be observed that sometimes even the original formulation is not a good shaving soap, something one finds in some artisanal soaps— particularly, it seems, those made with olive oil. The artisanal soaps I list are currently good; be careful in trying others and if possible buy and test a sample.

Shaving cream

Shaving creams come in a wide variety, including unscented creams (for example, Truefitt & Hill Ultimate Comfort) for those with sensitive skin. If your skin is sensitive, as described above in "Skin sensitivities," it's a good idea to test any new product—cream, soap, aftershave, etc.—before using it on your face.

Cyril R. Salter Mint is a great summertime shaving cream and their Vetiver is intense—as it should be. J. M. Fraser's Shaving Cream[98] has a light fragrance, creates a good lather, is curiously effective at softening the beard, and gives a fine shave. Taylor of Old Bond Street Avocado has received high praise[99]:

> I couldn't agree more on the [Taylor's] avocado. The scent is nice and light but not as luxurious as some others. The real value for me is the lubricity you described [from the avocado oil (persea gratissima) in the formulation] along with zero irritation. The absence of coloring and heavier scent additives I think is what drives this. In my opinion, this benefit makes this the ideal cream for a newbie, which I am.

Taylor of Old Bond Street, Truefitt & Hill, and Geo. F. Trumper are the "three T's" of fine English shaving creams and soaps. Castle Forbes is another fine shaving cream, available in lavender, lime, or cedarwood. It's pricey (perhaps better to receive as a gift than to buy). Luxury creams are also available from D.R. Harris, The Gentlemens Refinery, and others.

Some artisanal soap makers also make shaving creams so look for shaving creams on their sites. Al's Shaving specializes in shaving creams, and those he makes are highly regarded and definitely worth trying; he offers a 7-cream sampler that's quite nice. Em's Shave Place makes a lathering shaving cream that comes in a plastic dispenser bottle: you squirt some onto your brush and then build the lather—it produces a fine, thick, moisture-laden lather. The dispenser makes this an ideal shaving cream for those who shave in the shower, though I use it frequently and I shave at the sink.

You can buy shaving creams in a tube or a tub. Generally speaking, the price per ounce in a tube is twice what it is for the same cream in a tub. Some excellent shaving creams, though, are available only in a tube—Proraso shaving cream (from Italy) is one example. Other "tube only" shaving creams are Musgo Real (from Portugal), Speick (whose excellence far exceeds its modest price) and Tabac (both from Germany), and men-ü (in the UK and US). The men-ü cream is particularly concentrated so only a tiny bead is required.

Some shaving creams are non-lathering but produce fine shaves. Even though non-lathering, I find a damp brush is a better applicator than my bare hand. For creams such as these, no or very little water should be added, though the cream is applied to a wet beard. Nancy Boy shaving cream[100] is as good as any shaving cream I've used, and the signature fragrance is wonderful. The cream itself is highly protective and lubricating. Cremo Shaving cream, Anthony Logistics, and Baxter of California are also good nonlathering creams.

Loading a brush—and indeed, getting a lather—is easier for shaving creams than for soaps, probably why novices prefer creams. The loading method depends on whether the cream comes in a tube or a bowl. (As noted above, Em's Shave Place sells shaving cream in a pump bottle.)

Shaving cream in a tube

The general advice is to use a lump of cream about the size of an almond, though a beginner might start with more—say, the size of a Brazil nut. As noted above, men-ü shaving cream is concentrated: use a bead the size of a kernel of corn.

The shaving cream is then placed on the brush or smeared onto your cheeks to begin lathering on the face, or placed in a lathering bowl for those who use that method to work up the lather.

Shaving cream in a tub

You can dip out a lump of cream and use it as described above, but I generally just twirl the wet (but shaken out) brush in the tub of cream to coat the tips with shaving cream, which I then use to build the lather. This requires a soft shaving cream, and the dipping/twirling should be done with care so that you do not scoop up too much shaving cream: you want a total amount about equal in volume to an almond/brazil nut.

Some shaving creams, though, are quite firm—soap-like, almost, and those I load as I load a soap, described in the Soap section below: briskly brushing the cream with a wet brush. Coate's Limited Edition shaving cream and Figaro shaving cream are examples of harder shaving creams.

Again, the building of the lather can be done on the beard or in a bowl. I definitely prefer to build my lather on my beard. I encourage you to experiment (as you've no doubt noticed) and try both methods from the beginning.

Shaving cream lather using a lathering bowl

To produce lather with shaving cream when using a lathering bowl, put the dollop of cream in the warm bowl, take the slightly wet brush (not too wet: you can add more water, but you cannot remove water), and use a motion that's more than stirring but less than whipping to work up the lather. (If you whip too vigorously, you'll get a lot of lather, but it will be unprotective because it contains too much air. You want a stiff, dense lather that contains water more than air.) The rapid stirring motion will create a thick, creamy lather. Too much water makes a lather that's bubbly and runny rather than dense.

Because shaving creams can produce quite a bit of (unprotective) lather even if you use too little shaving cream, you should experiment to make sure you're using enough—thus the note above for beginners to try a dollop the size of a Brazil nut instead of an almond. Then, as you gain experience, cut back on the amount of shaving cream until you find the right proportion. The lather should be dense enough—and contain enough water—to do a proper job.

An illustrated on-line guide[101] shows one method of lathering with a cream. In this guide, he uses water from a hot-pot (probably distilled water—I use hot water from the tap, but my water is relatively soft).

Shake water from the brush, so that the brush is damp and not wet, and then add driblets of hot water to the brush as you develop the lather. (If you use the sink-full-of-water method, just dip the tip of the brush into the water.) This produces an abundant and substantial lather that's just wet enough.

Shaving cream lather by lathering directly on your beard

This method seems much easier to me and not so finicky with the water—plus the feel of the lather is a better guide than the look of the lather.

- **For cream in a tube**, I squirt out the traditional almond-sized amount (except note that men-ü shaving cream requires a smaller amount) and smear the cream on my (wet, washed) beard on each cheek, then use the wet but shaken out brush to spread the cream to coat all my beard with a thin layer of shaving cream.
- **For soft cream in a tub**, I shake out the wet brush and twirl it in the tub to coat the bristle tips with the shaving cream, then take that to my (wet, washed) beard and brush to coat my entire beard with a thin layer of shaving cream.
- **For firm/hard cream in a tub**, follow the soap procedures below.

Continuing with the soft-cream method, whether from tube or tub, dip the tips of the brushes bristles in water or (what I do) run a driblet of water into the center of the brush and brush the shaving cream that coats your beard, working the water into the shaving cream and the shaving cream into the brush. This will begin the lather formation. As you add water to the brush and continue to brush on your beard briskly, the lather will build. Take your time with this: you want not only to create a good lather but also to work the lather (with its load of water) into the beard to continue the softening. You may at first add too much water—making practice lathers provides the necessary experience quickly—but if you add water in small amounts, you'll easily get a fine lather. Still, in doing practice lathers, try adding too much water to see what happens. The brush itself holds plenty of lather for a multi-pass shave.

Shaving soap

Shaving soap is a nice (and cheaper) alternative to shaving cream. Initially I found shaving cream much easier to use, but as I learned how to make good lather from soap, I found that I prefer shaving soap to shaving cream and now seldom use the latter. (I do have relatively soft water, important for soap.)

The "three T's" (Geo. F. Trumper, Taylor of Old Bond Street, and Truefitt & Hill), well known for their shaving creams, also make triple-milled shaving soaps, as does D.R. Harris, whose soap makes an exceptionally good lather. Another favorite from Britain is Mitchell's Wool Fat Shaving Soap[102], occasionally difficult to lather. (As noted above, try a few drops of Trumper Skin Food or glycerin on brush or puck if you have problems with MWF—or try a distilled-water shave.) Tabac[103], Dovo, and Gold-Dachs Rivivage[104], all from Germany, are fine shaving soaps. Klar Kabinette is a very nice, rose-fragranced, inexpensive German shaving soap that comes in 500 gram (1.1 lb) packages containing two bars: cut off a chunk to fit your soap mug or bowl. Klar Seifen, from the same maker, is more expensive but an extremely nice shaving soap—and Klar Seifen Klassik aftershave is also a favorite.

As mentioned above, Virgilio Valobra[105], an Italian company, makes a wonderful soft, bitter-almond-scented shaving soap; it comes in a standard-sized bar but is the consistency of clay so that you mash it into a mug or bowl. Vitos Red-Label (better than the Green-Label variety) is another Italian soap and is tallow-based and the same soft consistency as the Valobra. Vitos comes in 1-liter bars (and is a tremendous bargain): you simply tear off a wad and mash it into a bowl or cup.

Otoko Organics makes an extremely interesting, skin-friendly shaving soap with ingredients not found in other soaps—like soya emulsifiers. It makes a fine, stiffish lather. BruceOnShaving has a good review[106] of this unusual soap, which so far is sold only in Australia (but can be ordered online).

Institut Karité shaving soap (25% shea butter, like their shaving cream) is an exceptionally good shaving soap from France. Essence of Scotland makes "Sweet Gale,"[107] whose ingredients include bog myrtle, honey, mixed spices, cedarwood, and Aberfeldy single-malt Scotch whisky. The fragrances of honey and scotch remind me of a Rusty Nail cocktail—a pleasant association.

Some other exceptional commercial brands—those that produce for me a particularly rich and creamy lather—include Fitjar Såpekokeri (but note the ingredients include Sodium Lauryl Sulfate (SLS); some skin conditions react poorly to this, but for me it's a terrific soap), Martin de Candre (an amazingly rich soap—note that the lid is purely for shipping and should be discarded in use so the soap can dry between shaves), Creed's Green Irish Tweed (spectacularly expensive, but a superb soap), and Dr. Selby's concentrated shaving cream (which works like an excellent shaving soap).

Using soaps handmade by artisans can be a particularly pleasant luxury—they make fine soaps in a range of fragrances much broader than what a traditional soap company can offer. On the other hand, unless the artisan understands shaving and shaving soaps, an artisanal soap can be terrible—some seem simply to add some clay to bath soap, hoping to get shaving soap. (You don't: you get a bath soap with clay in it.) The mark of a bad shaving soap is that the lather, if you can get any, is both sparse and short-lived: by the second pass, the lather's gone. Be especially wary of soaps based on olive oil. If you get a bad shaving soap, just use it as a bath soap.

I have bought and tried soaps from these vendors (included in the Appendix) and found them to be quite good; experiment carefully with others.

- Al's Shaving (focus is shaving creams)
- Em's Shave Place
- Ginger's Garden
- Honeybee Soaps
- Kell's Original
- Mama Bear
- Mystic Water
- Nanny's Silly Soap Company (in the UK)
- Prairie Creations
- QED
- Queen Charlotte Soaps
- Saint Charles Shave
- Scodioli
- The Shave Den
- The Strop Shoppe

If you have skin sensitivities, get samples and test as previously described. Some with sensitive skin have reported that some soaps have too much in the way of essential oils. I've heard that about some soaps from Kell's Original, Mama Bear, QED, and Scodioli, so from those in particular you may want to buy samples if your skin is sensitive. Most of these vendors provide unscented versions as well as a great range of fragrances.

Some artisanal vendors offer a full range of products—beyond shaving soaps—and those products are worth exploring. Some of these soaps are really exceptional. I particularly like soaps from Queen Charlotte Soaps, Mystic Water, and Strop Shoppe. And their ingredients are wonderful. Strop Shoppe, for example, whose soaps make a particularly rich lather, lists the ingredients as:

> Ingredients: Stearic Acid, Glycerin, Coconut Oil, Palm Oil, Rice Bran Oil, Fragrance. May contain Sunflower Oil (used as a substitute for Rice Bran Oil when needed).

And, of course, you can make your own shaving soap. You can find various recipes on the Web, but one easy way is to use Bramble Berry's melt-and-pour shaving soap base[108]. Other recipe links are in the endnote.

Soap in mug or bowl

The first—and critical—step is to load the brush with enough soap to create a good lather. Some use a damp brush, some (including me) prefer a wet brush.

Damp-brush method: Squeeze water from the brush, then brush the soap for 30 seconds to load the brush. Move to the beard or to a lathering bowl—and I believe that men using this method often favor a lathering bowl—and add small amounts of water until the lather is where you want it. The common rationale for this method is that water can be added, but it cannot be removed. On the other hand, this method is (for me) much too finicky: painfully slow and roundabout. I recommend (and use) the wet-brush method.

Wet-brush method: Wet the brush fully, hold the tub or mug or puck of soap on its side over the sink, and for 30 seconds brush the soap briskly and also firmly—if the brush has a 2" loft, get the top of the handle to 1" from the surface of the soap. At first, water and loose, sloppy lather will spill into the sink, but keep brushing. Soon you'll see real lather forming, but continue the brushing for 30 seconds or until you see no large bubbles: you want the brush fully loaded with soap. (Not all brushes spill water: I used two Simpson brushes recently, a Chubby 1 Best and a Duke 3 Best, following the wet-brush method described, and the water from the brush mixed right in with the lather.)

You could use a bowl for this method as well, but I move the brush to my (wet, washed) beard and continue to work the lather up and into the stubble. I have never once found that I have too wet a lather, but sometimes I do need to add a little water because the extended loading picks up a good amount of soap. Adding water is easy: I run a driblet of water into the center of the brush (or you can dip the tips in hot water) and then work that into the lather.

In either case, making good lather is a matter of experience, so get as much experience as quickly as you can by making practice lathers. Try loading for the full 30 seconds, then make a lather with a 25-second loading period, then a 20-second loading period. Try starting with a lather that's clearly dry (i.e., a damp brush fully loaded with soap) and adding just a little water as you work the brush with the soap. (This can be done on the beard or in a lathering bowl.) Work in the water each time and then feel the lather between thumb and forefinger. At first, it will be almost sticky. Then, as you hit the sweet spot, the appearance of the lather will change, and it will feel slick. As you continue adding water, you'll find that soon the lather becomes sticky once more.

After several practice lathers using the same soap each time, you'll know the look and the feel of a good lather. You can then transfer this knowledge to other soaps, which may require a different amount of water for the sweet spot. After you know it, the sweet spot is clear—some say the lather "explodes" at that point, but the lather doesn't so much increase in volume as change state.

You'll note the continuing theme in shaving: the need to experiment to find what works well for you. Guidance (as from this book) can be helpful, but the best teaching and the truest test are found in your own experience, and practice builds experience efficiently. The more you practice, the better you'll become. Fairly soon, you won't need to time the loading: you'll know from experience when your brush is sufficiently loaded and whether to add water or not as you work the lather.

Em's Shave Place has more information[109] on lathering from both soaps and creams. Razor-skipping when you shave (razor head not gliding smoothly across your skin, but seeming to "stick" and then skip) might be due to hard water, but it also might be a problem with the lather. If you switch creams and soaps a lot (trying different samples, for example), you may not find the sweet spot for a particular cream or soap and be using too much (or too little) water.

Use the brush to work the lather thoroughly into your beard. You need only enough lather to fully cover the whiskers—that is, the lather need not be deep on your face. Keep the lathered brush (whether using cream or soap) handy. After each pass, rinse your beard (it does not need to be a thorough rinse—a splash of water will do) and relather your beard prior to the next pass. Lather is always applied to a wet beard. Each pass with the razor requires a lathered (and thereby lubricated) face.

Take a look at this excellent on-line tutorial[110] (with photos). I don't bother with putting water on the soap—I experimented with doing that and with not doing it, and it made zero difference that I could tell. But definitely do your own experiments: that's how you learn what works for you and what doesn't.

A video referenced earlier[111] shows the quick creation of lather. The brush is the Kent BK8, a soft brush that some presume is "not good for soap." The video clearly shows this notion is false. The soap is Kent shaving soap (same as Mitchell's Wool Fat shaving soap), and the lathering bowl is the Moss Scuttle. And the water is soft. The BK8 can be used for face lathering, but the BK4 is a better size for that.

If the lather is inadequate (thin and sparse), the cause is almost always that either the brush is insufficiently loaded or the water is hard. Insufficient loading can be from brushing the soap too lightly or for too short a time.

I have found that horsehair brushes work best (for me) for making a good, creamy lather. Boar brushes also work well (and particularly require extended loading), and better as they become broken in. Badger and artificial badger make and hold a good amount of lather, but with these the novice has a tendency to stop loading the brush too soon: try for 30 seconds initially.

Soap in a shave stick

A shave stick is simply shaving soap in stick form. These are pleasant to use if you have a normal beard: the stubble scrapes the soap from the shave stick when you rub it against the grain of your beard. Two types of beards present a challenge. A beard that's sparse and soft, as for a man just beginning to shave, will not rub off enough soap to make a good lather. However, as shown in the (terrific) movie *The Dam Busters* (1955), a shave stick can also be used as an extraordinarily thick puck of small diameter, with the shaver loading the brush by brushing the end of the stick, as if loading from a puck.

In contrast, a heavy, thick, cheesegrater beard will scrape off *too much* soap, so that the lather will be soap-heavy and require a *lot* of water. Men with this sort of thick, tough beard should rub the sick only on part of their beard—say, on the chin and around the mouth—and then work the lather up there with the brush and gradually work it into the rest of the beard. Another possibility, suggested by cathartica, is that men with very tough beards rub the stick *with* the grain instead of against the grain.

Shave sticks are great for travel: they require no lathering bowl and their physical format is compact. Except for Queen Charlotte Soaps, the artisanal vendors mentioned above also make shave sticks.

Some quite good soaps are available only as shave sticks (Arko, for example), and men who do not like to use shave sticks on their beard can use the stick as a puck, as described above, or grate the stick and press the gratings into a mug or bowl to be used as a regular puck. I haven't tried this because I enjoy using a shave stick in the traditional way of rubbing it on my beard.

A variety of shave sticks are shown in the photos. On top, from left: D.R. Harris, La Toja, Boots, Tabac, Irisch Moose, QED, Mama Bear, and Honeybee Soaps. On bottom: Valobra, Erasmic, Lea, Palmolive, Speick, De Vergulde Hand, Arko, Mennen, and Wilkinson.

Some shave sticks don't have a container and

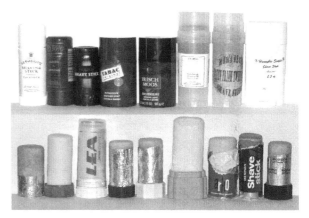

are simply cylinders of soap, perhaps wrapped in foil or paper. These can be packed for travel in a tall plastic prescription pill bottle. All the shave sticks shown produce an excellent lather.

You can also make your own shave sticks from any easily-melted shaving soap (*not* triple-milled soaps). Take the shaving soap puck, melt it, and pour it into a shave stick container. It's a simple process[112], but be careful not to get the soap too hot, lest you lose or alter the fragrance. And if you want, you can carve a shave stick from a puck of soap. Obviously, you can also make your own shave sticks from the Bramble Berry melt-and-pour shaving soap base.

As noted above, in using a shave stick you load your beard with soap, rather than your brush. After washing and rinsing your beard, rub the stick against the grain of your wet beard—over the entire beard for a normal beard, over just the Van Dyke area (or with the grain) for a tough thick beard. I have never found it necessary to wet the shave stick, but you may wish to experiment with using the shave stick dry and then on another shave using it wet to see which works best for you. Wetting the stick seems to help when the humidity is exceptionally low (centrally heated houses in very cold weather, for example).

Once your beard is well soaped, begin brushing briskly all over your beard with your wet shaving brush. Lather will appear, as if by magic. Continue brushing until the brush is fully loaded with lather, which also works the lather into your beard. Normally, a lathering bowl is not used with a shave stick, but it certainly would be possible. Try it and see if you like it.

Superlather

A "superlather" uses both shaving soap and shaving cream—best seen in an online video[113]. Use a lathering bowl and begin to build the lather from a shaving soap—but also add a dab of shaving cream and work that into the lather as well. The result is a particularly slick and dense lather.

StraightRazorPlace has a particularly good and detailed tutorial on making a superlather, illustrated with photographs[114].

Another way to generate superlather: use a shave stick to apply soap to your prepped and wet beard, then twirl the brush in shaving cream and lather on your beard. The soap, together with the shaving cream, produces a thick, luxurious lather. I like QED's Lavender shave stick and Em's Shave Place Lavender shaving cream. A Fresh Lemon shave stick from Honeybee Soaps works extremely well with the J.M. Fraser shaving cream. A shaver who doesn't particularly like either the l'Occitane Cade shaving soap or shaving cream alone found that the two work spectacularly together in a superlather.

EIGHT

The blade

THE blade and razor are the key components of the shave itself (as distinct from the prep). Novices tend to focus more on the razor because it's more obviously interesting than the blade and also much more expensive. Yet the comfort and smoothness of your shave, once your prep and technique are good, will be about 80% from the blade and 20% from the razor.

High-quality double-edged blades generally run 25¢-55¢ each in a pack of 5 or 10—the "Swedish" Gillettes (alas, now rarely found) were 90¢ apiece—and as low as 7¢-14¢ each if you look around for bulk lots—for example, on eBay or from blade vendors on-line. As noted earlier, Derby blades are now available on Amazon for $12.93/200 (with average blade life, that amounts to about $3.37 for a year's supply of blades), but Derby blades don't work for everyone. In fact, they don't work for me and seem tuggy. I prefer Astra Superior Platinum blades, which I got for 9¢ per blade. Blades come from Germany, Turkey, Pakistan, India, Japan, Sweden, Egypt, Israel, the UK, the US, Russia, Poland, and other countries.

With the right cutting technique on a well-prepped beard, the typical blade lasts about a week. Your own experience may well vary, depending on your prep, your beard, your skin, your technique, your razor, the brand of blade, the phase of the moon, etc. A range of 3-6 days is typical. There's no sense in trying to stretch a blade beyond its life—some blades will die gracefully, simply starting to pull and tug as they become dull, but others go out with a bang and start nicking. Change the blade as soon as the shave starts to suffer.

Double-edged blades cost substantially less than today's disposable multiblade plastic cartridges, which run as high as $3.50 each, and the usual rationalization for buying lots of delicious shaving equipment is that you'll be money ahead (eventually—sometime in the next 20 to 30 years) because of what you'll save on the blades.

Remember: the usual story is that blades are where Gillette makes its money—give away the razor, sell the blades, and over time, the total spent on blades is much more than the price of the razor. (The true story is more complicated[115].) Certainly with multiblade cartridges costing what they do, double-edged blades save you money immediately and over time save a lot.

Finding the right blade

DE blades offer a couple of surprises. The first, already noted, is how *smoothly* and *easily* the DE blade cuts through the stubble compared to a cartridge razor—because using a cartridge means pulling 3-6 blades through the stubble simultaneously, so naturally the effort required is 3-6 times what is needed to pull a single blade through stubble. (Keeping a cartridge razor on the face while cutting against such resistance seems to require much more pressure than a DE razor needs: thus cartridge shavers develop a bad habit of pressing hard—a habit that can cause serious problems with a DE razor.)

A second surprise for DE novices is how greatly brands of DE blades differ in sharpness and smoothness. One shaver wrote:

> Just started wetshaving 2 weeks ago… have only used Merkur blades since they came with the razor.
>
> Leisureguy suggested I order a 5-blade sampler with plan to try the blades in this order: Merkur -> Israeli -> Derby -> Gillette -> Feather
>
> I rec'd my sampler yesterday and tried the Israeli this morning… WOW!!
>
> I could not believe the difference. My best shave so far by leaps and bounds. The razor was gliding across my face and by the 3rd pass it was the closest most comfortable shave I have had yet.

The third—and greatest—surprise is how shaver responses to any given brand of blade vary so widely. For example, Treet Blue Special, a brand that is sharp and smooth and produces a highly satisfying shave for some (including me) seemed dull and tugged fiercely for others. The same surprising difference sometimes occurs when you use the same brand of blade in different razors: a blade that's uncomfortable and works poorly in one razor can perform quite well in another, presumably because of small differences between the two razors in blade angle, exposure, and the like.

Since a blade that someone else likes may not work for you (or your razor)—and a blade that they hate might work fine for you—trying blades yourself is the *only* way to find your own "best blade(s)." View skeptically comments such as "this blade is excellent" or "this blade is terrible." Those reflect *the speaker*'s experience. You *must* use the blades yourself to actually know how the blade will work *for you*.

The unpredictability of a shaver's response to any given brand of blade is mysterious but readily observed: Each brand has some who love it, some who hate it, and some who are indifferent. Some brands have a preponderance one way or the other, but even if only a few hate (or love) a brand, what if you are one of those few? You can't use the brand statistically: "I love this particular blade 60%, and hate it 35%, and am indifferent 5%."

With an individual shaver and a particular blade, the judgment is 100%, whether love, hate, or indifferent. So each individual shaver has to try multiple brands to find the brand(s) that work best for him, rather than simply pick those that are (statistically) popular. And if a shaver never ventures beyond the popular (and better-known) brands, he may never find his ideal blade.

If it were not like this—if all shavers responded in the same way to a blade (which many novices believe is the case and simply ask "Which blade is sharpest?" as if that would be the best blade for them)—then there would exist only one brand of blade: THE blade. Perhaps it would be sold in different colors of packages, or with different decorations printed on the blade, but everyone would use it because it is the universal "best" blade.

But life is not like that, and so blade sampler packs were developed to allow a shaver to try a wide variety of brands through one purchase.

I suggest that you get a large sampler pack, along with as many brands as you can buy locally. Samplers that have only one blade per brand are useless: don't get those. Initially, you won't be trying all the blades—that's for later. At first, try just one brand. (Guys who like Derby blades will suggest a Derby; guys who like Personnas will suggest that; and so on. Just pick a brand.)

If that brand seems to work reasonably well, stick with it. If you have trouble (usually "trouble" means the blade tugs at the whiskers rather than cutting easily, but sometimes it means nicks or skin irritation), even though you're being careful with your prep, blade angle, and razor pressure, try a different brand. You may have to try three or four. But as soon as you find a brand that seems to work, *stick with that brand* and don't try another brand until you're consistently getting good shaves—smooth, nick-free, and predictable. This may take from one to three months, and in some cases more.

This is important: if you keep changing blades as you learn, you will find it difficult to develop your groove. It would be foolish if you used a different make of tennis racquet each set while you were trying to learn tennis. It is similarly foolish to skip from brand to brand to brand of razor blade, one shave each: if you did that, you would never really learn any brand of blade and whether it actually does work well for you.

Experienced shavers all recommend that, once you find a brand that seems to work reasonably well, be faithful to that brand until your technique is solid and you are good at doing a basic double-edged safety-razor shave. At that point, your prep is solid: you can easily create an excellent lather, and when you bring blade to beard, your beard is fully wetted and as soft as it's going to get. Moreover, when you shave, you're not hesitant: your strokes are smooth and efficient, and you seldom encounter a nick or any skin irritation. You enjoy your shave, and the result is a smooth face and a jolly outlook.

At this point, you're ready to find whether your shave can be improved. If you followed the suggestion above, you already have the sampler pack with the greatest number of brands. If not, get it now. Then start working your way through the pack. The goal is to find a blade that produces a significantly smoother, easier, and more comfortable shave, with no nicks or burn.

Why explore?

Of course, once you're getting good shaves, you might think, "Why try another brand? This one's doing okay. Better just to stick with it." Indeed some (probably most) shavers do stick with the first brand they encounter that gives them a passable shave. I've read comments along the lines of "This brand tugs a lot, but when I'm finished, I have a good shave, so it's a good blade." Or, in the case of guys who ask, "Which blade is sharpest?" and someone tells them that Feathers are, they go with that brand and stick with even if they find they suffer chronic razor burn and constant nicks—they assume that is just what DE shaving is like.

It shouldn't be. If you find that a blade tugs a lot or feels harsh or seems to scrape, and you're pretty sure you use good technique (covered later), it's not a good blade for you. Shaving is about the process as well as the end result: both should be pleasurable, and the blade is a mission-critical component.

By continuing to explore even after you're getting good shaves with a particular brand, you might find a blade that takes your shave to a whole new level. That's most likely to happen if (a) you've so far been shaving with a limited range of blades—the usual suspects are Merkur, Astra, Personna, Derby, and Feather—and (b) the best brand for you is not one of the common brands.

It may happen, of course, that your best brand may be the brand you're already using—though, if you haven't tried many different brands, it's unlikely: the range of blades is quite large, you'll discover. And it may be that none of the new brands you try will really astonish you with the excellence of the shave. But it's likely that you'll find a blade better than you imagined possible. You have much to gain and little to lose from such an exploration.

My experience started with trying the usual beginner blades. The Merkurs were horrid (though they are excellent for a few), the Israelis and Derbys tugged too much where my beard was tough. The Swedish Gillettes were good but expensive. The Feathers were sharp but I kept getting unpredictable nicks—some experienced shavers can't use Feathers at all.

But when I started trying a wider variety of blades, I found a brand of blades that did indeed make me say, "Wow!" It cut smoothly, easily, and never produced a nick or any sign of irritation. It was the Treet Blue Special, a carbon-steel blade that (at the time) cost 2¢ each—and (of course) it does not work well for everyone. But I was one of the lucky ones. What a fine shave it gave!

I naturally recommended it to others, and some had the same reaction as I: shaving nirvana! Others, however, probably thought I was crazy.

Don't try just that one brand, though: it probably won't be a transcendent blade for you—though it might. To maximize your chances of hitting a lucky strike, try as many brands as you can. If you're lucky, you'll find a blade whose excellence is beyond that of any blade you've tried before. At the very least, you can enjoy some inexpensive exploration and learning. Blade acquisition disorder is the least costly of all the shaving-related acquisition disorders, much cheaper than acquisition disorders for razors, shaving creams, brushes, shaving soaps, aftershaves, and the like.

How to explore

To begin your blade exploration, load a new brand in a familiar razor and shave, using the good technique that you've mastered. If you get a terrible shave, discard that blade and try another blade of the same brand—it may have just been a bad blade. If the second blade of the brand also gives you a terrible shave, discard it and mark that brand off the list: it's obviously not for you. (Note that this means that sampler packs with only one blade per brand are useless: if the blade you try is bad, it may be a dud, but there's no second blade to try.)

EXCEPTIONS: If you have more than one razor, try the blade in another razor before you give up on it. A blade that's terrible in the HD might be wonderful in a Gillette Super Speed and vice versa. Also, note that some blades seem dull for the first shave or two, until the coating that covers the edge is worn away. Sputnik, Dorco 301, Tiger, and Crystal, among others, are like this.

Here's a careful and methodical approach. Call the blade that so far works best for you the "best blade."

1. Shave for a week with the current "best blade." This sets a baseline.

2. Shave for a week with a new brand of blade (unless it fails the test of two terrible shaves).
3. If the new brand is the better of the two, it is now your new "best blade": go to 2 to try another new brand.
4. If the new brand is not better, go to 1.

By using this approach you're always comparing just two brands: your best so far and a new brand. That makes the comparison easy, and by always starting the comparison with a week shaving with your "best blade" (so far), you not only get a break from testing, you get a fresh reminder of what a blade that's good for you feels like before you try the next new brand.

Sometimes two different brands are almost equal in quality. To compare those, use each brand on alternate days so you can get a closer comparison. On the other hand, you might want to move faster. Since at this point you're an experienced shaver with good technique, you will usually know after three or four shaves whether you like a new brand of blade or not. This greatly cuts down exploration time—but still it's a good idea to return periodically to your current "best blade" and shave a while with that to re-establish the standard. And remember that some brands will not shave smoothly for the first shave or two—your own response to a blade should be your guide, but try for three shaves at least before you decide a blade is dull.

As you explore, you'll find blades fall into one of three classes:
1. **Some won't work for you.** For such a brand, write a note on why it's not good for you (too dull, nicks too frequently, irritates your skin—whatever), put the note and the remaining blades of that brand in an envelope, write the brand name on the envelope, and put it aside. After six months or a year, try the brand again to see whether things (your prep, technique, razor, etc.) have changed and the brand is now good for you. If it's still not your cup of tea, pass the blades along to someone else—for him, they could be a "best blade".
2. **Some will work fine**—just as good as the blade you've been using, or perhaps even a little better. Add these to your rotation for variety.
3. If you're lucky, **one or two will make you say, "Wow!"** These blades are, for you, truly exceptional: they shave so smoothly, so easily, so readily that it's as though you've not really had a great shave before.

My own current best blades are: Astra Superior Platinum, Wilkinsons, Zorrik, Polsilver, Iridium Super, Gillette 7 O'Clock SharpEdge, and Lord Platinum.

"Swedish" Gillettes are excellent but are no longer made, and the same fate has befallen Iridium, Astra Keramik, the Treet black carbon-steel blades, and others. Blade brands can vanish at any time, so when you find a brand that you like a lot, consider buying a large supply while you can. Right now Gillette is making a major push to move third-world shavers to cheap cartridges (more profitable than blades, plus lock-in to the Gillette brand), and any particular brand of double-edged blade could be discontinued without notice.

Once I liked Feather and Tiger blades, but then I decided that they were too ready to nick for no reason. They seemed like a high-powered but unstable motorcycle: great performance but unpredictable. And yet I'm now finding that Feather blades work quite well in the new premium Feather razor.

It's the same story with Gillette 7 O'Clock SharpEdge blades (not to be confused with the 7AM brand). They were so sharp that I could not comfortably use them—not erratic, just very, very sharp. I set them aside and continued with other blades. By the time I got around to trying them again, they were perfect. It's just as your music teacher told you: daily practice improves your skill.

With a microscope you can see the actual differences in the edges of different brands[116]. Microphotographs of the edges of several common brands show clear differences. The Treet Blue Special clearly has a well-sharpened edge—still, it doesn't work for some shavers, though it works extremely well for others (including me). A series of reviews[117] on ShaveMyFace of different brands of blades has a microphotograph of the blade being reviewed. The reviews are helpful, though how well the blade shaves for the reviewer may not be the experience that you or I would have. Again: different shavers can respond quite differently to the same brand of blade—an idea that's extremely difficult to internalize.

It's worth noting that cartridge shavers get few choices of brands and types of blades—many fewer than DE shavers have, who can also choose among various kinds of steel (carbon, stainless, tungsten stainless, etc.) and various kinds of coatings (platinum, chromium, Teflon, etc.). Cartridge razors have to make do with the very few varieties available—and what's available may for you fall far short of the shave that a "best blade" can deliver.

Carbon-steel blades

Some blades (Treet Blue Special, Treet DuraSharp HiTech Steel, Treet Classic) are made of carbon steel rather than stainless steel. I know from using knives (and reading about straight razors) that carbon steel can take a sharper edge than stainless steel, but carbon steel does tend to rust. So if you find you like a carbon-steel blade, you have three choices:

    a. Use a new blade for each shave (they're cheap).
    b. Dry the blade after each use (*not* by rubbing it with a cloth but, for example, by rinsing it under hot water and then shaking it well or using a hair dryer).

c. Easiest: After shaving, rinse the razor in hot water, give it a good shake, swish the head in 91% or 99% rubbing alcohol, and then put it in a rack to dry. The alcohol displaces the water and then evaporates, leaving the blade dry so that it doesn't rust. (This technique also works in hard-water areas to prevent mineral deposits along the blade's edge as the hard water evaporates.)

I go with option c., using an inexpensive 99% rubbing alcohol I buy at the local Safeway supermarket. If you do this, use a squat, wide-mouth jar that originally contained a food product: the mouth is large enough to accept the razor head, and a commercial jar's lid opens/shuts with one quarter-turn.

If you use alcohol for your straight or DE razor, simply dip the razor in the alcohol and remove it: never let it rest there for long: it will discolor steel and ruin resin handles. Avoid bleach like the plague: it destroys metal quickly.

One shaver reported that the oil remaining on the blade's edge after completing the Oil Pass (described below) kept the edge from rusting.

In the Great Depression (long before stainless blades arrived), small hones were made to resharpen double-edged blades, which at that time were all made of carbon steel. You can occasionally find such hones on eBay. They don't work on coated stainless blades, and I don't think they're worth the effort on carbon-steel blades. Razorpit.com does sell a kind of plasticized strop to clean the edge of the blade without removing the blade from the razor: it does seem to work, especially if, when the blade becomes tuggy, you turn the blade over in the razor, retighten the head, and strop the other size. But given the price of blades (and of the Razorpit device), this does not seem to me to be cost-effective.

More about blades

Blades are generally printed with the manufacturer's name and other information, so the two sides—top and bottom—look different. You can put the blade in the razor with either side on top: it makes no difference. Since you use both edges of the razor as you shave—when one side of the razor has collected enough lather, you switch to the other side for a while before you rinse the razor—the blade's two edges thus are worn down simultaneously.

Merkur manufactures both blades and razors, and so they naturally include their own blades with the razors they sell. Unfortunately, Merkur blades for the majority of men (and thus probably for you) are terrible. If you get a Merkur razor, blade exploration (and a blade sampler) is particularly important.

Some novices wonder whether turning the blade over after a few shaves will make it last longer. It might, but given the price of blades, it doesn't seem to be worth the effort. Moreover, it's a good idea to avoid handling the blade, whose cutting edge is delicate and easily damaged. But try it if you like: experiment.

Some, as previously noted, find that a given brand of blade works well for them in one razor, but not in another. For example, a very sharp blade might work well for them in a Gillette Super Speed, but not in a Merkur HD. The practice of shaving is a on-going series of experiments that you perform.

If you find a brand harsh, you can pull each edge of a new blade through a wine cork before using the blade ("corking" the blade). This tames the blade's edge while leaving it still sharp enough to shave. My own view is that it's better to find a brand that works for you without corking. Moreover, given how easily a blade's edge is damaged, the result of corking can be a blade that's much the worse for it—and for you. So my own inclination is to explore more brands of blades before I try corking a brand I have. Others like to do the corking. You decide for yourself which you want to do.

I do want to provide one blade warning. I had a chrome Merkur Slant Bar that provided me with lovely, perfect shaves even when I used it with a Feather blade—and never a nick. So I decided I had to have a Slant Bar in gold. I sold the chrome Slant Bar, got the gold, put in a new Feather—and Nick City! I was aghast. I tried again the next day: still a lot of nicks. I was despondent, but eventually I tried a new Feather blade, replacing the one in the razor.

I got a perfect, lovely shave, and not a nick. So it was a bad blade. I had read of this, but that was my first experience of it. I probably would have immediately tried another blade if: (a) it wasn't my first shave with the new razor (thus blaming the razor instead of the blade, still thinking that all blades of a given make were the same); and (b) it wasn't the first time I had ever encountered an instance of a bad blade (it's rare); and (c) I hadn't panicked, thinking I had just sold the one Slant Bar in all the world that would work for me.

Lesson learned: if you have a bad shave with a new razor, try changing the blade. And if you then have a bad shave with the new blade, try a different brand of blade. Don't jump to the conclusion, as I did, that the razor is the problem. Experiment.

Blade disposal

Razor blades remain quite sharp even when too dull for shaving, so disposal requires some care. Plastic blade dispensers usually have a "used-blade" compartment on the bottom for safe disposal.

If your brand lacks the dispenser, use a special receptacle for used blades rather than simply throwing the blades into the trash—razor blades can all too readily cut through plastic trash bags and into the hands lifting the bag.

Proper disposal of sharps is *always* worth doing with care. States and cities often have laws and ordinances regulating the disposal of biohazard sharps, and blades belong to this category. (Call your local waste management company or municipal department for more information on appropriate sharps containers and where to dispose of them.)

You can easily find commercially made disposal safes for razors—some pharmacies even provide free sharps containers. The Feather Blade Safe[118] works well, and Pacific Handy Cutters makes a wall-mounted blade bank[119].

But it's also very easy to make quite a good blade safe. Take a small can—for example, a small can of evaporated milk or tomato juice—and drain the contents by punching two small holes in the top. Wash out the can, using the two holes. Then turn the can over and, using a hacksaw or a thin Dremel blade, cut a slit in the side, just under what was the bottom and is now the top. Make the slit just wide enough to admit a double-edged blade.

The can then sits (upside down, with the two small holes you made in the top now out of sight at the bottom) and you discard the blades through the slit, just under the now-top. When the can is full, a tap of a hammer permanently shuts the slit: an opaque, unbreakable, metal blade safe with no lid to open. I use this and after more than six years of six-day-a-week shaving it's only now becoming full. Note, however, that this homemade container, though safe, may or may not meet local requirements for a sharps container.

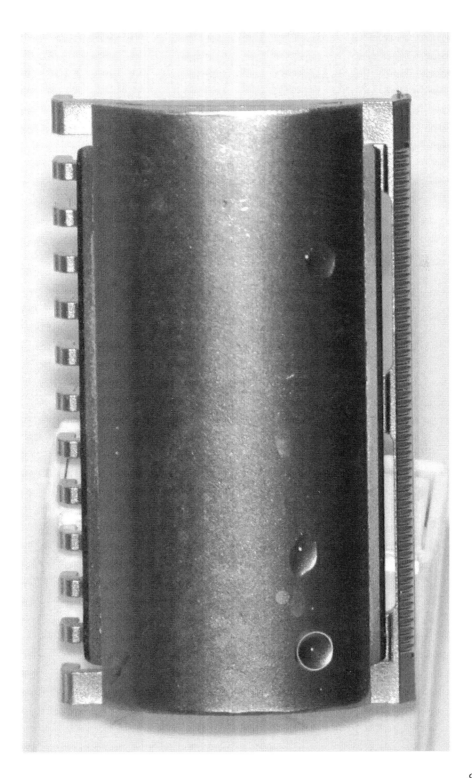

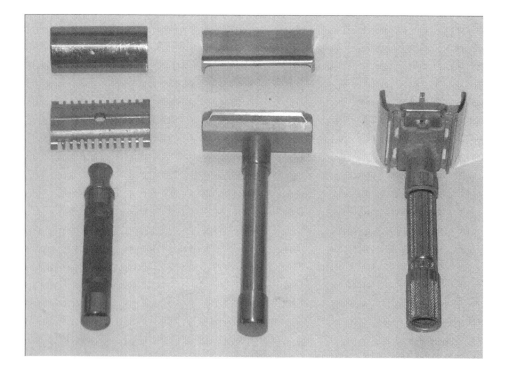

NINE

The razor

THE focus of this book is the safety razor (see photo opposite). Before the safety razor, there was the straight razor, but once the safety razor arrived, it quickly displaced the straight[120]. Safety razors are sometimes called "handles," an odd locution since the razor *has* a handle: the new terminology leads to (for example) talking about the handle of the handle. In this book, I'll use "razor" to the refer to the razor and "handle" to refer to the handle.

The blade is the very center of the safety razor system, and it was the blade that gave King Camp Gillette his opportunity and the challenge: to manufacture a sharp, disposable blade from thin, stamped steel. The safety razor holds the blade and presents the edge with a specific exposure and angle. The safety razor can be:

Three-piece (like the early Gillette razors and the Edwin Jagger DE8x series: top, baseplate, and handle) – *left opposite*: a Gillette NEW (introduced in 1930); this type is the easiest to pack since it's lies flat once disassembled; it's also the sturdiest;

Two-piece (like the Merkur Futur, Hefty Classic ("HD"), Progress, and Slant Bar: top and baseplate-handle) – *center opposite*: a Pils razor; or

One-piece (like the Merkur Vision, Gillette Super Speed, and other twist-to-open (TTO) razors: twisting the knob at the bottom one way opens butterfly doors for changing blades, the other closes them to grip the blade for shaving) – *right opposite*: a Gillette Fat Boy. One-piece razors are the most fragile and prone to damage if dropped: lots of moving parts and insecure joints.

With a three-piece razor a beginning shaver will sometimes put the razor together with the baseplate upside down, which results in the razor either not cutting at all—or if the shaver persists, in producing a bloody harvest of nicks. If the guard is scalloped on one side, those scallops are on the top side of the baseplate and face the cap, away from the handle. Inspect the razor closely before removing the baseplate, and when putting in the blade, make sure the baseplate is right-side up before tightening the cap.

In the photo at the right are two baseplates from Edwin Jagger razors. The baseplate at the top is right-side-up, and the side shown faces the cap. The baseplate at the bottom is upside-down, and the top of the handle fits into the circular depression in the bottom of the baseplate.

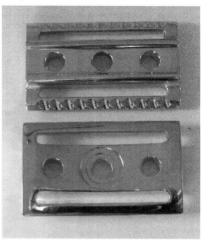

To load a three-piece razor: place the cap upside-down in the palm of the non-dominant hand, drop/push a fresh blade over the studs for proper alignment, then place the baseplate (scalloped edges facing the cap) on the blade and screw the handle onto the threaded stud projecting through the baseplate.

Two-piece razors, with the baseplate and the handle joined into a single unit, must solve the problem of how to attach the cap to the baseplate-handle. The usual attachment is threaded; the challenge then is how to turn the threads while the cap stays in a fixed orientation with respect to the baseplate-handle. The common approach (used in the Merkur HD among others) is to have a threaded shaft that can rotate independently inside the hollow handle, the shaft turned by a knob at the bottom and engaging the threads from the cap's central protrusion. Generally a friction ring that allows easy rotation prevents the shaft from falling out. The friction ring allows the shaft to be removed for cleaning.

Another approach, used by the Pils shown and by the iKon SK9, is to attached the handle to the baseplate with a bearing so that the handle rotates independently. In this case, the action is much like a three-piece razor.

A third approach, seen in the Merkur Futur, is to do away altogether with a threaded attachment (and the corresponding requirement for easy rotation) and instead attach the cap to the baseplate with a snap-on connection.

Em's Shave Place also has a good explanation (with photos) that explains these three types of razors[121].

In razors using double-edged blades, the blade is held between the cap and a baseplate, with only the edge exposed. As the razor is tightened to grip the blade, the cap bends the blade over the slight hump of the baseplate, making the edge rigid and presenting the edge at a specific angle, which differs slightly for different razors. (Single-edged blades, like those used in Gem razors and Schick

Injectors, are rigid to start with because they are made of thicker steel, and thus do not have to be bent in the razor's grip as do thin, double-edged blades.)

Novices sometimes fail to tighten the razor sufficiently after inserting the (double-edged) blade. The cap must be seated *firmly* onto the blade, to bend it over the baseplate and hold it securely. (The Futur's design cleverly finesses this error: the top *snaps* on, so if it's properly in place, it's holding firmly.)

The question is sometimes raised: *how* tight should the cap be? So, a little scenario. You're going on a picnic. Just before you pack the jar of pickles, you open it and eat one. Then you put the lid back on and put the jar on its side in the basket. *That* tight: tight enough so the jar won't leak and the lid will stay on, but not so tight that your mother, wife, or girlfriend can't remove the lid at the picnic.

The reason to tighten the cap carefully is that an insufficiently tightened razor becomes a bloodletting threshing machine. This is particularly an issue with one-piece (TTO) razors. In the Fat Boy, for example, resistance is encountered just at the point where a final quarter-turn is needed: that last bit of resistance is similar to that of a lock nut—easy tightening until the end, then more torque required for the final quarter turn until the razor locks. Do that extra quarter-turn.

A razor stand is optional: I store my razors lying on their side on a shallow shelf. You can buy a stand for a single razor from various places, or you can use a test-tube rack for multiple razors: the razors in current use. A razor stand or rack is useful because you want the razor out where it can dry after you shave. Do not put it into a drawer—it won't dry so well and the blade's 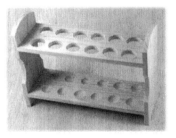 edge is more likely to be damaged in a drawer (much as you do not put your quality kitchen knives in a drawer, but keep them in a knife rack). Turnabout's fair play: a blade whose edge you nick will nick you.

Handles

Three-piece razors generally use standard threads, so that one razor's handle can be attached to another's head: a "Frankenrazor". Some manufacturers of new stainless three-piece razors offer a choice of handles and even sell the handles separately. Handles are available from iKon, Pens of the Forest[122], Tradere, and Weber. A solid stainless Bulldog handle can greatly change the heft and feel of a razor whose original handle was much lighter, being hollow or made of resin. The difference in weight, diameter, knurling, and appearance produces a noticeably different shaving experience—and, of course, the same handle can be used on many different three-piece razors, illustrating another advantage the three-piece format has over the two-piece and the TTO: interchangeable parts.

The Merkur Classic head and the newer Edwin Jagger head are also available from Elite Razor in various handle materials: stone, resin, wood, and snakeskin (with clear plastic coating). I have two razors from Elite: a Merkur model (white quartz with gold lacings) and an Edwin Jagger model (red jasper). Both are *very* nice to use: the heavier weight makes shaving a dream.

Pens of the Forest, BadgerBrush.net, and Penchetta make razors with custom handles. Penchetta also sells kits for you to make your own razor.

Since handles are available for separate purchase, you can also buy a razor head by itself and combine it with your own handle—one you've made or a handle you've purchased separately—to make a complete razor. Edwin Jagger, whose new head design is excellent (and discussed later) does sells their razor head separately[123].

Smooth handles vs. knurled handles

Razors are commonly available with smooth handles—resin (faux ivory and faux ebony, typically), stone, wood, bone, and chromed metal. Since in shaving one's hands are often wet, you may think such handles could be slippery. Obviously, if the handle is wet *and* soapy, it will indeed be slippery, but soap is readily rinsed away. A smooth handle is slippery when soapy, but even a soapy knurled handle is slippery unless the knurling is extremely aggressive—more aggressive than on most razors. I tested a Merkur HD and a Gillette Fat Boy, which have knurled handles, and I found the grip was slippery when my hands were wet and soapy; when the soap was rinsed away, I had a secure grip with wet hands, as I do with wet (but not soapy) hands and a smooth handle.

Based on a poll I ran on the ShaveNook forum, a wet smooth handle presents no problem at all for 80% of shavers, though 20% do find that a wet smooth handle is slippery—particularly a chrome smooth handle—but for most the slipperiness declines over a week or two. The cause may be a polish applied to new razors that wears off in use, and perhaps also a difference in the shaver's skin contributes to whether the grip is secure or not.

I was completely unaware of this problem—I'm in the lucky 80%—until recently. I ran the poll after learning of the problem, and the result surprised me.

If you have a smooth-handled razor and you're one of the unlucky 20%, the simplest solution is to brush your wet fingers over the alum block; your grip on the razor will then be secure. A more complicated and less elegant solution is to wrap the handle with some non-slip tape or band or ring, but the alum block is right at hand, as it were, and it works, so that's what I recommend. And as noted, the problem in many cases diminishes over time as you use the razor.

Open-comb vs. safety bar

Some razors have a guard that is an "open comb"—separated teeth instead of a solid bar. Open-comb razors have the blade either resting on the teeth (the Merkur and old Gillettes) or just above the teeth (the improvement introduced with the Gillette NEW IMPROVED (1921) and used in later models). The safety bar is a solid bar that rides on your skin just ahead of the blade as you shave. A razor with a safety bar is often called a "straight-bar" razor.

The open comb was the original design, with the straight bar introduced later. The straight bar is easier to manufacture and it's less fragile. If you drop an open-comb, you're likely to bend a corner tooth. The straight bar does, however, squeegee away the lather, whereas the open-comb leaves some lather in place as the blade hits the stubble. In practice, however, the straight-bar razors shave perfectly well, despite pushing the lather away.

Some open-comb razors are designed so the blade rests directly on the comb—for example, the Merkur Hefty Classic Open Comb. In others, the design has the blade held above the teeth by a "coat-hanger" profile of the base plate—for example, the Gillette NEW, first offered in 1930 and still a well-loved razor, particularly the model with long, bent-over teeth instead of shorter teeth. The difference in design doesn't seem to matter: they shave equally well.

An open-comb razor has a different feel from a safety-bar, but you can get a good shave with either. Most men opt for the safety bar design simply because it's much more common. The quality of the shave is due mostly to the prep, the blade, and your technique, in any case.

Edwin Jagger razors

Edwin Jagger razors since 2010 use a new head design developed by Neal Jagger and the Müller brothers of Mühle-Pinsel.
Customer feedback on the new head has been excellent: it delivers a great shave and the new design is easier to clean. A novice occasionally makes the mistake of putting the razor back together with the baseplate upside down, which pretty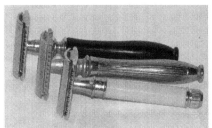
much ruins the shave. Note in the photo that the three Edwin Jagger razors have the scalloped edge of the baseplate as the *top* side, facing the cap. The new head

is shown on the razor in front, a DE87 model, which has a faux ivory handle. As you can see, the curved side of the baseplate is the bottom. The lined Chatsworth behind it and the Chatsworth with the faux ebony handle have a Merkur Classic head, which Edwin Jagger formerly used. That head is discussed in the Merkur section below.

Edwin Jagger razors come in a variety of designs and are solid performers worth considering[124]. The plating on the current models is heavy chrome, but if you're interested in gold plating, you can contact them for a special order. For your first razor, I strongly recommend one of the Edwin Jagger DE8x series.

The current Chatsworth models all use the new head design—those in the photo are older versions that I've had for some years. The Chatsworth models are appealing to those who prefer a longer handle—either for regular shaving or, as for bicyclists and swimmers, for shaving their legs. As noted above, for 80% of shavers the smooth handles present no problem even if wet, but if you find the handle is slippery, brush your wet fingers across an alum block and your grip will be secure.

Merkur's Classic head was for many years the standard; I myself began shaving with a Merkur 34C, the "HD." When I got my Edwin Jagger with the new head, it seemed fine—I had one of those "gradual awareness" experiences in which over the course of several shaves I went from mild acceptance of the new razor to a realization that it really was a marked improvement; it just took me a while to notice. I had to "learn" the new razor (with any new razor there's a slight learning curve that may take one or several shaves), but as I become more accustomed to it, I became more enthusiastic about its performance.

I recently did an inadvertent blind comparison[125] of the Merkur Classic head and the new Edwin Jagger head (used also on Mühle razors): I was doing a two-razor shave testing the smooth-handle situation, and I had assumed that both razors—an Elite Razor with a quartz handle and a Gerson (a rebranded Mühle Sophist) with a bone handle—had the Merkur Classic head (which Mühle, like Jagger, formerly used). I did the first pass with the Elite, and as soon as I began the second pass, I was surprised by the difference—and by how much better the Gerson felt: it turned out to have the new Jagger head design.

Feather razors

Feather, a Japanese company that makes extremely sharp blades (which, of course, do not work for some: YMMV), also makes razors. One particular Feather razor, the AS-D1, is notable for quality (and price). It's a three-piece all-stainless-steel razor—a simple design executed with extreme precision. While expensive, it's extremely comfortable and a pleasure to use. It also makes a nice gift item because of its presentation in a small wooden box, somewhat like a trophy.

Naturally enough, it works extremely well (for me) with Feather blades. It's the razor at the bottom of the three shown.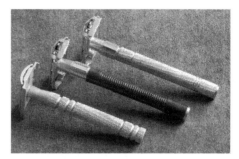

Feather also makes an inexpensive model, the Feather Popular, useful as a beginner razor. It is lightweight and shaves reasonably well and is the middle razor in the photo. An all-metal version of the Feather Popular is sold as the Diamond Edge brand, the razor at the top of the photo. That razor is included in an inexpensive beginner kit from Whipped Dog[126]. However, I highly recommend the Edwin Jagger DE8x razor for a beginner, though it costs twice as much. The Edwin Jagger is heavier, better made, shaves better, and will be a lifetime razor.

Gerson razors

I have but one, which my wife bought in Paris. It is a rebranded Mühle Sophist with a horn handle and shaves quite well. I know little about the line. I also have a Gerson brush, a good brush, but Gerson products are rare in the US.

iKon razors

Gregory Kahn has a small company in Thailand that has for some years offered stainless steel three-piece razors (and one two-piece razor, the SK9) in a variety of designs, both open comb and with a bar guard and—uniquely—with an asymmetric design: open-comb on one side, bar guard on the other.

iKon razors are well-made and distinctly *comfortable*. These razors are expensive but of extremely high quality. He regularly comes out with new models, so if you don't see one you like, keep an eye on his Web site.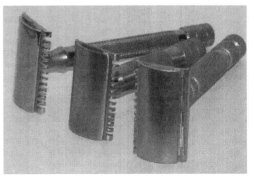

In the photo, the razor in front is the iKon OSS, one of his asymmetric razors; that in the middle is the S3S, a wonderfully hefty razor; and the one in back is the second iKon to come to market, and now discontinued: an open-comb three-piece razor. The SK9 is a two-piece design that, like the Pils, has the handle attached to the baseplate with a roller bearing so the handle rotates to tighten the cap. The iKon razors are stainless, but I did have the long-handle open-comb in the photo gold-plated (by Razor Emporium, which offers a plating service).

My initial thought about the asymmetric design was to use the open comb for the first pass and the straight-bar for the later passes. But as it turned out, both sides seemed to me completely comfortable and equally suited to the entire shave, including beginning and end, so I simply use it as a regular razor, using one side until it's full of lather, then switching to the other. I enjoy the slight change of feel during the shave, and the shave itself goes well.

Some, on looking at the asymmetric design, have suggested that the razor be modified to make both sides open comb. The thought had also occurred to me, but in using the razor I changed my mind. The two different guard formats give this razor a dual personality, and that's the idea for this particular model. (iKon is at work on other models that will be symmetric, but asymmetric razors seem to have a permanent place in the iKon lineup.)

The dual-personality aspect in effect gives the shave a new dimension: instead of shaving with a single razor-guard format, you have two in the same razor. You could, of course, switch back and forth between two different razors in your collection—in fact, Bruce Everiss describes in detail the technique of a three-razor shave[127]—but having two formats in one razor is convenient.

With the iKon asymmetrics, the two edge formats are "in tune," as it were: switching back and forth is not only comfortable, it's pleasant—like hitting one note and then a harmonious but different note: think of a drum solo played on a single drum versus one using two drums. The difference in the shaving experience as compared with a traditional (symmetric) razor is pleasant—it turns out that the two-format OSS provides a shave that (to me) is more interesting and richer than a shave with a razor that has just one guard format.

The market offers *many* razors whose two sides are identical. If that's what you want, you have an embarrassment of riches. But a single razor that provides, metaphorically, a three-dimensional shave unlike the two-dimensional ones delivered by symmetric razors? Those are rare: only the iKons so far.

Joris razors

Joris is a French make that offers top-of-the-line razors, some plated in palladium. The blade angle on the Joris heads seems to be markedly different from other razors I have (save for the new Mühle open-comb released summer 2011 and described below). I found these razors quite harsh until I got the advice to use a 20° angle of attack instead of the 30° angle commonly used with other razors: with this head, a shallower angle of attack removes the harshness that results from doing more scraping than shaving: to prevent scraping, reduce the angle of attack.

This reinforces the point that, whenever you get a new razor, you must do a certain amount of experimentation to learn how best to handle it—and quite often you must do some blade exploration as well: a blade that works well for you in one 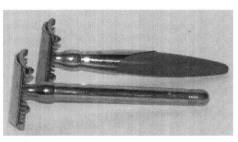 razor may not work so well in another—and vice versa. With the Joris I relied on the habits I had established with other razors: a mistake. Still, I ultimately decided that these razors don't work so well for me; YMMV.

Lord razors

Lord is an Egyptian company that makes a range of razor blades and also some razors. The three-piece Lord L6 razor is popular with beginners for much the same reasons as the Feather Popular: it's inexpensive and has a reasonably good head. The L6 does have two drawbacks. First, it is very lightweight, so maintaining the right pressure is more difficult than with a heavier razor, where the razor's weight can do the work. Second, the razor is light because the (long) handle is made of aluminum: not only light but also soft, so that its threads are easily stripped. Using a handle from some other razor for this razor is often a necessity rather than an option. I don't recommend this razor for that reason. The Feather Popular is a better choice as a beginner razor, but an Edwin Jagger DE8x is *much* better than either and is also a lifetime razor.

Merkur razors

Of razors still in production, the Merkur line, made in Germany, is currently the most commonly available. Though occasionally a problem may be encountered (typically, uneven exposure, with the razor exposing one edge of the blade more than the other), your dealer will replace any problematic razor with a new one. Starting with a Merkur razor is still a common route for the beginner—nowadays the 180 model seems to be frequently chosen—but the new Edwin Jagger/Mühle head in my experience shaves better and more easily, so I highly recommend that a novice start with one of those. I did begin with a Merkur (the

HD model was the common beginner choice of the time), but that was some years before Edwin Jagger and Mühle came out with their new head design.

Some Merkur razors are available in either chrome- or gold-plated versions. There's no difference in performance, only in appearance. Merkur razors are normally shipped with Merkur blades, which work well for few.

Merkur non-adjustable razors

Non-adjustable razors have a fixed blade angle and exposure. With no adjustment to consider (and tinker with), the novice shaver has one less thing to worry about—for example, if the shave is bad, the novice doesn't have to figure out whether it's his technique that's at fault or the particular setting of the adjustable razor (or both). Thus the best "starter razor" is non-adjustable.

Classic

The Classic line of Merkur razors all have the same head geometry—only the handles differ. Thus they all shave the same, though the different handles do indeed give them a different feel.

Hefty Classic (the "HD")

The HD boasts solid construction, a thick handle, and a good blade exposure and angle so that it removes stubble efficiently without being harsh. Nonetheless, some novices find the HD too aggressive for them and prefer a vintage Gillette Tech or Super Speed or a Weishi razor, all milder than the HD.

Classic

The same as the HD, but with a slimmer handle. Again, a good starter razor, lighter than the HD. One benefit of this razor's three-piece design is that the razor is flat when disassembled, making it easy to pack for travel.

Long-Handle Classic

If you like a long-handle razor, this would be a good choice. I found that, for myself, the long handle was unhelpful and even seemed to get in the way—but the long handle makes this a good choice for shaving one's legs.

180

The Merkur 180 serves as a beginning razor for many, but I do note a fair number of men who started with the 180 comment on how much better they like their second razor (a vintage Gillette, for example, or the Edwin Jagger, or some other razor). Based on those reactions, I feel ambivalent about the 180.

1904

This Classic's handle has a somewhat ornate design based on earlier razors. It was my second razor, and I continue to like it a lot. The little knob at the end of the handle is perfect when shaving against the grain. It would be nice if it were available in gold. I went for a replating, but found that the 1904 is plated in chrome, and replating over chrome apparently presents 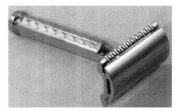 technical difficulties, so my 1904 remains as it was, still a satisfying razor.

38C

The Merkur 38C has the Classic head, but a longer, heavier handle with a fine, deep, spiral engraving. Unfortunately, due to its weight, I found the razor difficult to hold with wet hands—it tended to twist because of the spiral engraving. A chequered engraving or a smooth handle (as on the Futur) would have been better for me. Some shavers rest the end of the handle on the little finger to avoid the problem and love the razor, but I tried it twice, and both times I had to sell it.

Slant Bar

The Slant Bar is an amazing razor with an intriguing history[128] and provides effortless, smooth shaves when used with a sharp blade that works for you. On the other hand, in polls for the best razor for a beginning shaver, *no one* recommends that a novice start with the Slant Bar. But when one has learned good technique, the Slant Bar seems tailor-made for the combination of thick, wiry beard and sensitive skin—a combination, I'm told, that particularly afflicts the red-haired. In my opinion, **a Slant Bar should be your second razor**.

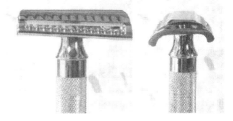

The Slant Bar works best with a sharp blade. I recommend you try the Slant Bar only after you're getting consistently good shaves with your current safety razor—that is, your technique (maintaining the correct pressure and angle) is solid. Once your technique is polished, you can move to a new level of ease and closeness by using a Slant Bar. A poll I ran on ShaveNook.com showed that about 70% of those who try a Slant Bar love it—though it doesn't work for about 7%. Still, when it works, it works very well indeed[129]. If it doesn't work initially, put it aside a few months and then try it again: often the problems do not reappear.

The Slant Bar is handled *exactly* as a regular safety razor. The difference in performance is due not to any manipulation on your part (as in the "Gillette slide"[130]) but to the slant of the blade. Rather than chopping directly through each whisker, the slanted blade *slices* through the whisker when you pull the razor normally. The photo above from Em's Shave Place shows the slant clearly.

Compare the action of the Scottish Maiden and the Guillotine: both are designed for decapitation, but the Scottish Maiden's blade is straight across—delivering a chop as it falls—whereas the Guillotine has an angled blade, to slice instead. In practice, the Guillotine proved far superior because the Scottish Maiden's blade, even when sharp, tended simply to crush the victim's neck.

I believe that very fine stubble, when fully wetted and cut short, similarly tends to be "crushed" by a standard straight-bar razor: rather than being cut, the fine stubble is simply pushed over, and this results in a rough patch once the stubble has dried and regained its strength. The slanted blade, in contrast, does not push directly against the stubble, but slides through it, slicing it before it can move: the slanted blade does not meet (or produce) the same resistance as the head-on attack of a straight blade.

Shaving stubble on the neck is often a challenge because of grain weirdness and the way the straight-bar razor pushes directly against the stubble (and the stubble against the skin). The Slant, slicing smoothly through the stubble, encounters no resistance and evokes no push-back.

The Slant Bar's way of holding the blade does the slicing automatically. Again: you do not wield the Slant Bar any differently than you would, say, a Hefty Classic. Shave with light touch and proper angle and don't even think about the fact that it's a Slant Bar (or Hefty Classic). The way the razor is constructed will take care of the cutting. Again: *light* pressure with the Slant Bar.

The 39C "Sledgehammer" has the Slant Bar head on the same heavy spiraled handle as the 38C, and presented to me the same problem as the 37C: a strong tendency to twist in the hand. I didn't like it; others do.

Merkur adjustable razors

Adjustable razors allow the shaver to change the angle and/or amount of blade exposed. I recommend you do not get an adjustable as your first safety razor for reasons stated above. Still, some novices do start with an adjustable and succeed.

The key to success with an adjustable razor is to start with the lowest setting—the setting that has the least blade exposure and the flattest razor angle. Then you advance the setting from shave to shave as needed to get a good shave. What you seek is the *lowest* setting that produces a good shave, *not* the highest setting you can stand. The settings usually start with "1" as the lowest setting, with higher numbers for longer, thicker, tougher stubble.

Despite this advice, a surprising number of new shavers, through misplaced pride and machismo, will start with the razor at its highest setting and get an amazing razor burn along with a harvest of nicks. Avoid that mistake.

Progress

The Progress adjustable is a two-piece razor, unusual in that the cap has only one correct orientation. A line stamped on one end of the cap must be placed above the triangle stamped on one end of the base. It's a delight to use, though the correct angle for this razor differs quite a bit from the HD angle. But whenever you pick up a new razor you have to learn the proper angle for it—this is called "getting used to it" and is much like getting a feel for how best to hold and cut with a new kitchen knife.

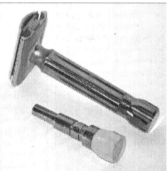

The Progress is well designed—a hefty, chunky razor that feels good in the hand. It's a favorite of many shavers, though some complain of uneven blade exposure. One shaver noted a cure[131]: press down on the top (with your fingers hooked under the base, like a syringe) and then tighten the knob. This prevents blade slippage as the tightening occurs.

The photo above shows a Progress and, beside it, the original knob that tightens the head. A replacement knob by iKon Razors is on the Progress. Since I have a gold Progress, I had the stainless knob gold-plated as well.

Futur

The Futur is a good safety razor, heavy and substantial. The Futur is particularly aggressive, so by all means start at setting 1, and gradually work your way up until you get a satisfyingly close shave. For me, that was at 1.5, though eventually I've moved to 2.0. Some guys have started with the setting at 4 or even higher and then regretted it bitterly. I found that I got the smoothest shave with the Futur if I took careful note of the procedure for all safety razors: to rest the cap on the skin being shaved, rather than the guard. Try different angles with it to find the angle that works best for you.

Some have found the Futur's adjustment to be stiff. One shaver offers this advice[132]: "First remove the blade, then set the head to position 6. Now press the blade carriage and the bottom of the head together, hold against the spring pressure, and unscrew the handle with your other hand. Now that you have it completely stripped down, put some silicone grease on the threads and reassemble in the reverse order of the above. This still leaves the adjustment heavy due to the spring pressure but makes the action a great deal smoother."

The clip-on top is, I think, a clever design: if you've snapped the top in place, the blade is properly gripped. No need to wonder about how firmly you should screw shut the top. Others don't like the clip-on so much. If you are changing blades, it's highly advisable to do so with dry hands and a dry razor. A slip can produce a cut.

The Futur is available in a matte finish or a shiny finish in chrome or gold. The 80/20 split described earlier doubtless holds for the Futur: 80% will not find it slippery when wet; the other 20% can use the alum block trick.

Vision

The Vision (technically the "Vision 2000") is even more massive than the Futur. Some have reported problems with the Vision, apparently from internal hard-water deposits. Sometimes the problems are severe and prevent adjustment. If you encounter a problem, it's handy to have what amounts to a Vision user's manual[133], though it's obvious that the Vision was *not* designed for easy field-stripping. 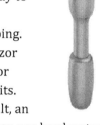 The best approach is prevention: making sure to clean the razor after each shave and, if you have hard water, soaking the razor periodically in a 1:4 vinegar water solution to dissolve deposits. Because disassembly and reassembly of the Vision are difficult, an ultrasonic cleaner (described later) is extremely helpful. (If you use hard water, think twice about buying a Vision.)

The Vision is heavy and, using a good blade that suits you, you can clearly hear it cutting the stubble, a sound like the distant rampaging of an elephant through brush. I do greatly enjoy using the Vision.

Mühle razors

I have a couple of Mühle razors (pictured) that I like a lot: a Sophist—the one with the porcelain handle (very cool)—and an R-41, an open-comb razor with spiraled handle. The R-41 is not so heavy that the razor tries to twist in my hand. 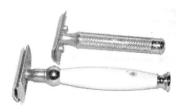 Both razors do a fine job, and Mühle makes fine razors and brushes.

In summer 2011 Mühle changed the R-41 head. The new head has a very different angle of attack from the old and requires a very shallow angle to avoid scraping the skin, which makes the head feel harsh. I found that using the razor was not enjoyable: harshness was a threat on every stroke. I sold it fairly soon, but some like it because they have heavy beards and appreciate the extremely aggressive attitude of the 2011 R41. However, for a heavy beard I would recommend a Slant Bar instead.

Parker razors

Parker razors a few years ago were of indifferent quality, but the company has consistently worked to improve their razors, using heavier-gauge metals and improving quality and design. I now have a couple of Parker razors, and the shave is perfectly reasonable—and certainly many use a Parker as their first razor. The 92R has seemed good, the 99R was harsh—but they're the same head. I still don't quite have a handle on the Parker line. Given that the Edwin Jagger is in the same price range, I recommend that brand instead.

Pils razors

Pils, a German company, makes a line of shaving gear in a "modern-machine" aesthetic: unadorned machined surfaces. 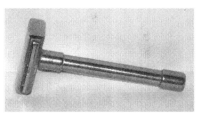 Their stainless razor, for example, has only the word "PILS" stamped on the base of the handle; otherwise, not a letter or numeral on it: no manufacturer logo, no patent number, no model ID.

It is a good razor, beautifully made, and it shaves extremely well, due in part to the design of the head, which rounds sharply just above the blade's edge, thus stretching the skin just before the blade passes. It's a two-piece design, and (as in the iKon SK9) the handle is attached to the baseplate with a roller bearing so the handle itself rotates readily. The first stainless model was prone to rust spots under the cap, due to a problem with a supplier, but those models were recalled. And, of course, the other models, being brass, never had the problem.

Tradere razors

Tradere is a new razor manufacturer, currently offering a handle (sold by itself) and an open-comb razor. This razor, like the 2011 Mühle R41, requires a very shallow angle. Some easily master the angle and like the Tradere razors very much[134]. It took me a while to learn, but with practice I got it. The new straight-bar Tradere, in contrast, is extremely comfortable and quite efficient. (I tested a prototype; the razor is soon to be released.)

Weber razors

Weber, another new manufacturer, is based in Missouri. Currently two models are available. The first is a razor whose head has a DLC (Diamond-Like Carbon[135]) coating, a smooth, abrasive resistant coating, often used on drill bits, dies, molds, and high-performance engines. The razor is extremely comfortable and shaves well, with the DLC coating feeling smooth against the skin.

Their other razor—currently my favorite razor—uses "ARC" (Advanced Razor Coating), a chromium-based coating commonly used on medical devices. The ARC Weber not only shaves with superb comfort and smoothness, it somehow manages to easily shave the flat-lying stubble under my chin. The Weber web site explains the special properties of the two coatings.

Weber has other razors planned, so check their site. Many shavers have reported that by their third shave, the Weber has become their favorite razor.

Weishi razors

Weishi makes good-quality razors, but they are so mild in their shaving action that I can't use them. A Weishi would work as a razor for a beginner who has a light beard—a beginning shaver, for example. Manufacturing quality is good; it's the mildness that makes it not work for me.

Vintage razors

There's great satisfaction in shaving with a vintage razor, particularly one that your father or grandfather used, and many vintage razors deliver an excellent shave. Vintage razors can be found from time to time at local flea markets and antique stores. Also, elderly relatives, garage sales, eBay, and the Selling/Trading threads in the various shaving forums are all good sources. If you go the vintage route, it's better to buy via the Selling/Trading threads or through reddit's Shave_Bazaar rather than through eBay. Sellers on the shaving forums know razors and sell razors that will work—many eBay sellers don't know razors and will unintentionally sell razors that are not shave-ready (missing parts, bent head or guard, etc.). On the other hand, you're more likely to find an underpriced treasure from a seller—on eBay or at a garage sale—who doesn't know razors. Examine carefully any photos posted by an eBay seller. Look for misalignment and also any signs of worn plating, which often is seen on the cap.

Gillette safety razors abound on eBay. BadgerandBlade has a good post with photos showing some common Gillette razors[136] you might encounter, and a reference site[137] gives detailed information on how the production dates of Gillette razors are coded.

Sometimes you will receive a vintage razor that is damaged or bent, so inspect carefully any that you buy before using them. This does not necessarily mean that the seller sold a defective razor: if the razor shipped to you is not properly packed (in a sturdy box, for example), it can be bent during shipment. This happened to one razor I bought on eBay. So if the razor arrives only in a padded envelope, inspect it carefully—it may require a little corrective bending. You may want to request shipment in a box.

As with most things in shaving, preferences in razors vary by shaver: what works well for one person will not suit another. Still, several vintage razors—the Super Speeds, the Fat Boy, and others—generally get high praise.

Occasionally, a used razor will arrive with a blade in place. *Do not use that blade*—you don't know where it's been. Start with a new blade, fresh out of the package. Also, vintage razors will occasionally arrive with a package of old blades. Don't use them: the edges will be rough due to oxidation. Use only new blades that you've purchased.

When you buy a vintage razor, you frequently must clean it, and cleaning instructions are provided below. Some vendors, though, provide shave-ready razors, fully cleaned and sterilized.

Gillette

Tech

The Tech was made from 1939 through the 40's. It's a three-piece razor and gives a mild shave. In a poll of "best razor for a novice," the Tech came in third, just after the HD and the Super Speed. These are quite common—Gillette made millions of them—and they are generally inexpensive on eBay.

Super Speed

The Super Speed is the second most recommended razor for a beginner. It is less aggressive than the HD and slightly more aggressive than the Tech. It's a TTO (twist-to-open) razor: one piece with silo doors that open to admit a new blade.

Aristocrat

Gillette used the name "Aristocrat" for several different razors, including a gold-plated version of the Slim Handle adjustable described below, but the best (for me) is the 1940s version: a gold TTO razor, slightly more aggressive than the Super Speed. It's a favorite of mine. It's shown on the cover of this book.

Fat Boy and Slim Handle

The Fat Boy and the Slim Handle are two common Gillette adjustables. The lowest setting is 1, the highest (most aggressive) is 9. Start at 3 and adjust the setting as needed to get the shave you want. Some like the Fat Boy, which was version 1.0 of the Gillette adjustables, others prefer the Slim Handle (version 2.0). The head geometries differ, thus the correct shaving angles also differ. On the Web you can find excellent disassembly instructions for the Fat Boy[138].

Super Adjustable

The Super Adjustable is the last adjustable Gillette made. It has a black resin handle and is available in a nickel-plated version and a gold-plated version, and with a long or short handle. I have recently discovered that this is a very nice razor indeed. Those with a metal baseplate are best—the very last version used a black plastic baseplate.

Lady Gillette

A long-handled, non-adjustable TTO razor designed for women. The handle comes in pink, blue, or gold[139]. Although marketed to women, men also like the razor. Any long-handled DE razor would offer the same advantage for leg-shaving as the Lady Gillette.

Wilkinson

Wilkinson is a British company, and the popularity of Wilkinson double-edged blades in the US is what prompted Gillette to move into making the first multiblade cartridge. Wilkinson continues to make double-edged blades, along with razors and shaving soap (so-so) and a shave stick (good).

Wilkinson Sword Classic

The Wilkinson Classic[140] is in current manufacture as a low- priced entry razor, rather more substantial than most. It has enough heft t o shave well, though one shaver recently reported that the same blade (Astra Superior Platinum in his case)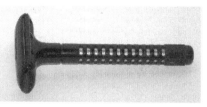
that shaved only so-so in the Classic shaved like a dream in his Edwin Jagger DE8x razor.

The "Sticky"

The Wilkinson "Sticky" is an exceptionally attractive razor, and it won a number of design awards. In addition, it gives a terrific shave, similar in some respects to a good Super Speed shave. They come up on eBay every now and then and are subject to fierce bidding. The name refers to the smooth plastic handle which is not slippery even when it's wet, but this turns out to be generally true.

Apollo Mikron

The Apollo Mikron is a vintage razor that was made in Germany. It shows up on eBay infrequently. It works somewhat like the Merkur Progress, and I really like the design. Pictured are the two I have. The best way to acquire one of these

jewels is to post a "favorite search" on eBay for Apollo Mikron and to be sure the search includes both the US and the European (German, in particular) eBay sites. Of the two pictured, the one in back, with the full-tapered handle, seems to do a better job.

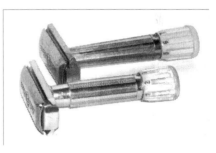

The resemblance to the Progress is so marked that I suspect the Progress may have been designed as a cost-engineered Mikron.

Eclipse "Red Ring"

Bruce Everiss posted on his (photo-rich) shaving blog a short history of this razor[141], made in the UK. It has a small magnet in the base of the handle to pick

up blades, a nice touch. It's an open-comb razor, but with a bar attached across the back of tips of the comb's teeth: this allows the open-comb action while offering excellent protection against bent or broken teeth. It's a very nice razor but extremely difficult to find.

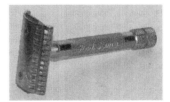

Single-edge razors: Schick & GEM

Two other razor options I should mention, because they're both very nice razors: easy to use and offering a comfortable shave—and they seem to work well for those who tend to get razor bumps. Both use a *single-edged blade*, made of thicker steel than double-edged blades. These two single-edged razors are the Schick Injector[142] and the GEM G-Bar[143].

Schick razors come in various models[144]. I have a G8, a J1, and an M1, and all do a good job with regular Schick blades, still readily available.

The GEM also has several models, but the one I call the "G-Bar" (with a circled G on either side of the handle) seems to give a better shave (for me) than the more common GEM Micromatic. Moreover, the G-Bar is usually available in excellent condition. The GEM razors are designed so that the blade is at the correct angle when the large flat head is held against the skin. This makes the razor good for head-shaving, since you can feel when the razor's flat against the skin even if you can't see it, and in that position the angle is correct.

Ted Pella Teflon-coated single-edged blades[145] work okay, but better are blades specifically made for shaving (Treet, PAL, and the GEM brands). Do **not** use hardware store blades made for utility knives: those are inadequate for shaving. Both the Schick (or "Schick-Eversharp") Injector and the GEM G-Bar are easy to find on eBay and generally run less than Gillettes.

Favorite razors

I do have certain razors that are more enjoyable than others. Apollo Mikron, Eclipse Red Ring, Feather stainless premium razor, Gillette Super Adjustable and NEW and 1940s Aristocrat, two Slant Bars (Merkur and a white bakelite model), the iKons, Edwin Jagger DE87, and—most of all—my Weber ARC.

I could add many more, but I tried (unsuccessfully) for a short list. Each razor seems to have its own personality, and I enjoy using them all. The Gillette vintage razors from the NEW to the Super Adjustable are particularly good.

Cleaning your razors

If you pick up an old razor on eBay or at a flea market or the like, you will have to clean it before using it. Moreover, your razors will also require cleaning from time to time as you use them—many, for example, clean the razor when changing the blade. If in your cleaning you notice hard-water deposits or soap scum, definitely try a distilled water shave as described earlier.

Hard-water deposits can make a TTO razor hard to operate. A one- to two-hour soak in room-temperature vinegar water (1:4 solution) loosens hard-water deposits to free the action, and a drop or two of mineral oil will lubricate the razor. Do *not* use 3-in-1 oil: it will turn gummy and worsen the problem.

Some are concerned about biohazard issues with vintage razors and want to take extra precautions to sterilize them. Here's a suggested procedure:

Step 1: First get rid of all encrustations and deposits (old soap scum, for example). There's no point in sterilization procedures if those are present. Open a TTO razor fully, and disassemble a three-piece razor. If the razor contains a blade, remove and safely discard it. If the razor is all-metal, you can soak it in room-temperature vinegar water (1:4) for an hour or two to dissolve or loosen hard-water deposits. Do **not** boil a razor in vinegar water: some razors use copper, which when boiled in an acidic solution will coat the razor with copper, turning a nickel plating yellowish.

After the soak, scrub the razor thoroughly with a toothbrush and a **nonabrasive** cleanser such as Scrubbing Bubbles or Bon Ami to remove any remaining deposits. A toothpick can help clear the grooves. Obviously, razors with handles of resin, bone, wood, or other such material will require greater care than an all-metal razor. Again: do not boil even all-metal razors in the vinegar-water, particularly a Gillette adjustable. In any event, boiling is not needed: this step is not sterilization, it's simply removing deposits on the razor.

If you have access to an ultrasonic cleaner[146], that works extremely well provided one uses an ultrasonic cleaning solution made for such cleaners. (Ad hoc improvised cleaning solutions of (for example) a little liquid detergent and household ammonia are sometimes used, but these are not so effective.) Note that ultrasonic cleaners of modest price generally have the transducer attached to the stainless tank via an adhesive and thus the contents should be at room temperature: in such cleaners the heat from hot water can weaken the bond between transducers and tank.

Good-quality ultrasonic cleaners are now available at relatively low cost. Look for a cleaner that's at least 50 watts. (Most ultrasonic cleaners for consumer use are 35 watts.) I have a Kendal CD-4800, a 60-watt cleaner that I found on eBay by searching for "ultrasonic". Fill the tank and run a full cycle to expel dissolved gases. Then put your razors in for one or two cycles, depending on how much cleaning is required. Afterwards a little polish may be needed to remove minor discolorations on smooth surfaces—for example, the razor's cap. The end result is a very clean razor, inside and out. If you know or suspect the razor is exceptionally dirty, let it soak in hot water with dishwashing detergent for an hour before putting it into the cleaner.

An ultrasonic cleaner can be used to clean jewelry as well—except do not attempt to clean opals, pearls, emeralds, or any stone with a chip or crack: the ultrasonic cleaner can destroy those, but it will not harm metal.

Step 2: Once the razor is cleaned, sterilizing can proceed. The extent of your efforts to sterilize the razor is a YMMV issue. The focus of sterilizing is the head of the razor: the part that comes into contact with skin, which may at some point be cut. Although in that case blood does come into contact with the razor head, note that in the process of shaving the razor's head is continually rinsed (to remove lather as it accumulates), which minimizes the chance that any blood was permanently deposited on the head.

Some will be satisfied at this point with rinsing and drying the razor. Some will want to rinse the razor or the razor head in rubbing alcohol (70% or higher). All-metal razors can withstand treatment (for example, boiling in plain water—*not* vinegar water) that would ruin a razor whose handle is resin, bone, wood, or other such material, but razors with those handles are likely to be three-piece razors; with those the head can be removed and sterilized alone.

Others with more concerns about sterilization may wish to let an all-metal razor (or the razor head from a three-piece razor: the only part of real concern) rest briefly in rubbing alcohol (though not for an extended period, which can discolor metal and ruin other materials) or run it through a dishwasher's sterilizing cycle or use a commercial sterilizing liquid such as Barbicide. Using bleach, particularly at high concentrations, can destroy the razor totally. Pictured is a Gillette Fat Boy that sat in bleach for just 10 minutes[147].

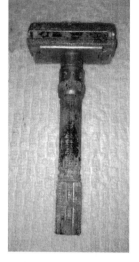

Some will simply not consider using a vintage razor under any circumstances, despite the fact that vintage razors are widely used with no problems reported. Certainly the risk from vintage razors seem much less than the risks associated with common hazardous sports—bicycling, for example—but each shaver must decide for himself his tolerance for risk.

I'm somewhat threat-insensitive to this sort of thing: I'm satisfied with the cleaning step and a rinse in alcohol, believing that the likelihood of a serious threat is low. I use many vintage razors regularly with no problems to date.

However, you should note that I have no professional expertise in sterilizing procedures: if you have concerns (and *especially* if you have a weakened immune system), do further research.

Art of Manliness has a good article on restoring vintage razors[148].

Maas metal polish[149] can help bring a shine back to your razor, but use only a tiny amount. Using Maas with a toothbrush can clean the chequered handles quite well. After polishing the razor, be *sure* to wash off *all* the Maas before shaving: it burns newly shaved skin. The problem with polish is that it is slightly abrasive, and the plating on most razors is thin: their manufacturers did not really design razors for decades of use.

If you have a silver razor, it's best to remove tarnish chemically rather than abrasively. Use a heatproof bowl deep enough to allow the razor to be totally submerged. Line the bowl with a piece of aluminum foil, put the razor on the foil, and sprinkle generously with baking soda. Pour in boiling water, let stand for half an hour, and the silver will be tarnish-free. I eventually had my own silver razors replated in rhodium, roughly the same color but non-tarnishing since it's an inert metal (of the platinum family).

Barbicide can help in cleaning. Immerse the razor for less than ten minutes—more may damage the plating—and then rinse the razor in water or in high-proof rubbing alcohol and let it air-dry.

If your razor is gold-plated, do not boil it. Let it soak for a long time in warm water, then cleaning it with Scrubbing Bubbles and a soft toothbrush. Boiling will remove the lacquer that protects the gold plating on some razors. The methods described above work well for routine cleaning, but a really good cleaning requires an ultrasonic cleaner, as described above.

Replating your razors

Gillette did not build their razors with an eye to long life: the expectation was that the buyer would replace the razor with a new model in a few years. So the original plating, being thin, was not very durable, wearing off in use—thus all the "brassing" seen on old razors. (Brassing occurs when the original plate, typically nickel, wears off to expose the underlying base metal, typically brass.) Replating can make an old razor look new.

Two vendors do replating: Razor Emporium in the US and Restored Razors in the UK. Both are listed in the appendix. You might also contact local jewelry stores to see whether they offer such a service or know a local replater.

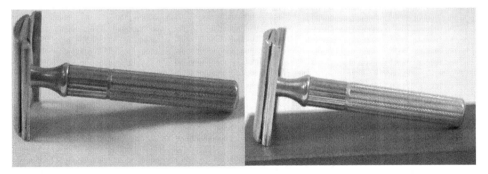

Above is a Gillette Tech that has been replated by Restored Razors— "before" on the left, "after" on the right. The plating in this case is nickel, the same as the original plating. Even so, the value to a collector may be less with the replating—but of course, the original razor with its worn plating was also of little interest to a collector. (Hard to please, those collectors.) Even so, you could decrease the value of a rare razor by replating it, so take that into consideration.

I went through my own razor collection and picked out those that both would benefit from replating and for which I felt a special fondness. Below is a set of my own razors that Razor Emporium replated in rhodium, a hard, silvery, inert metal. Because these were older and had some wear, I chose their complete refurbishing service rather than simply replating.

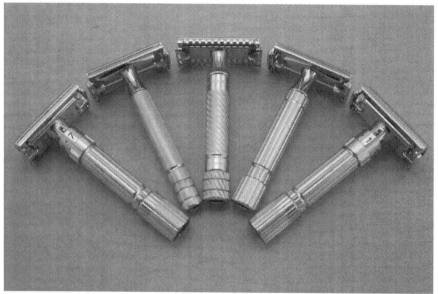

In the photo, from left to right: Fat Boy, Super Speed, English Aristocrat #22, President, Fat Boy, all made by Gillette. Since these five razors were replated with an inauthentic metal, collectors will not find the razors of value— but for the daily shaver, a freshly plated razor is much more pleasing than the worn original.

The cost of replating varies with the plating metal chosen: nickel, silver, rhodium, gold, or perhaps part plated with one metal and part with another (for example, part plated in silver, part in gold). The process takes a while, mainly because of the prep required, so it might be a month before you get your renewed razor returned.

The time that can elapse between shipping your razor off for replating and opening the box on its return may be longer than you expect. We're accustomed to a shipping delay when we place an order on-line: the time to ship from vendor to us. But consider that replating involves 4-6 shipping delays:

You ship to vendor

Vendor inspects, refurbishes, ships to replater

Replater inspects, preps, plates, ships to vendor

Vendor inspects – and at this point you may get more delays:

> Vendor finds flaw, ships back to replater

> Replater fixes flaw, ships back to vendor

Vendor ships razor to you

So you should be prepared to wait one month and perhaps (if a razor has to be redone) two. In my opinion, the final result was worth the wait.

A modern-day barbershop shave

A traditional wetshaver often wants to experience a good, old-fashioned barbershop shave: a luxurious relaxation under the ministrations of a practiced professional. The image many men carry into such a shave is of loads of warm lather whipped up with a wonderful brush, a hot towel, and then the skillful application of a straight razor that leaves a perfectly smooth face, ending with the wonderful glide of an alum block and then a splash of aftershave.

However, modern-day health regulations and current practice have changed that picture. No brushes will be used, for example, and no alum block: the barber is not allowed to use items such as those for multiple customers: health regulations forbid the practice to prevent infections. The lather comes instead from a lather machine, and an alum block is not to be seen.

And the hoped-for straight razor is likely to be a shavette at best (which uses disposable blades, replaced after every shave) or, more likely, a multiblade-cartridge razor, though at least a fresh cartridge will be used for each shave: no shaves with a two- or three-month old cartridge (as men often use at home).

One benefit of the multiblade cartridge razor is that it is easy to use and requires no training or learning or skill: anyone can use it from start as well as they will ever use it. So naturally one starts to think, "Why am I paying top dollar for this shave when the barber is using a razor that requires no skill whatsoever? I could do as good a job shaving myself at home."

And that's the sad bottom line: except in rare circumstances, a traditional wetshaver who uses a good brush, a good lather from a top-quality shaving soap or cream, and a good DE or straight razor is going to give himself a better and more luxurious shave than he would get in a modern-day barber's chair.

There are exceptions: the shaves at the Geo. F. Trumper and Truefitt & Hill shops in London are still top-notch, according to reports I've read. But your local barber? or even the average big-city barber? Not likely. The few shaving oases are well known to cognoscenti, but they tend to be rare and located in places like New York, Chicago, and other major cities and in vacation destination cities such as Las Vegas, though occasionally one reads of a tiny barbershop in some strip-mall that still manages to provide a wonderful and luxurious shave despite the setting. But such are increasingly rare as the older generations of barbers depart the business. And in any event, skills require continual practice to stay at their peak, and with so few seeking a barbershop shave, skills grow rusty and out come the multiblade-cartridge razors.

For most of us, the best shave is to be found in our own bathroom and at our own hands, using traditional wetshaving equipment, methods, and supplies.

TEN

Shaving the stubble

USING a safety razor puts *you* in charge, and going from a multiblade cartridge to a safety razor is like going from an automatic transmission to a manual: you can get better performance by being more in control, but you must learn how to use it, practice your technique, and pay attention to what's going on.

One point before you actually pick up the razor and put blade to face: Some shavers have one or more moles in the shaving area, and some moles are shaped so they are often cut. If you have such a mole, I *highly* recommend that you get it removed. It's a simple procedure and a dermatologist can do it in an office visit. Not only does it make your shaving life better, it also removes a mole that, being on your face, is constantly exposed to sunlight.

Pressure

The first variable you must control is *pressure*. With a safety razor, you must **not** use pressure to try to get a closer shave: pressure must be *light*, the razor and the blade doing the work—exerting additional pressure will cause problems (cuts, razor burn, lack of joy, etc.). As described below, you get a closer shave with more passes, *not* more pressure. Think of the razor as a little container of nitroglycerin and the head as a pressure switch. That should help.

To ensure light pressure, one shaver found that holding the very *tip*[150] of the razor handle with a two- or three-finger grip works well. This is an instructional grip, not intended for daily use, but try it for at least part of a shave to demonstrate to yourself how a razor with a sharp blade works well even with very light pressure. The most common error for the novice shaver is incorrect pressure—and so far as I know, it is *never* having too light a pressure.

Using too much pressure can be a general problem, or it can be localized: on the right side of the face for right-handers, for example, or on the neck, often a problem area because of the various curves. Or it can appear only on the against-the-grain pass when the razor is held upside down.

Symptoms of the problem are razor burn (face red and hot), small nicks, razor bumps, and skin irritation. If you think you're using too much pressure, try "negative pressure": holding off some of the full weight of the razor. A sharp blade will cut fine so long as it's pulled at the correct angle through the stubble. *Never* try to achieve a clean shave in one pass.

There are two reasons (I believe) for using too much pressure. First, getting a close shave with a multiblade cartridge requires pressure, so former cartridge shavers have a habit of pressing down. Indeed, some cartridge shavers, as the cartridge grows dull, continue to use it by exerting more pressure as they shave—a bad habit that causes serious problems when using a safety razor.

The second reason is that the shaver feels stubble when rinsing his face after the first pass and thinks he must not have used enough pressure. *Not so.* There *will* be stubble after the first pass—that's why you do multiple passes. The key is *progressive stubble reduction* over multiple passes: at least two, generally three, and sometimes four (explained below). Each pass leaves less stubble.

In particular, you want the stubble reduced as much as possible in the initial passes before you try an against-the-grain pass.

Blade angle

Besides pressure, the key variable in using the safety razor is *blade angle.* Try this: put the head of the razor against your cheek, the handle perpendicular to the cheek and parallel to the floor. Gradually bring the handle down toward the face as you make a shaving stroke, pulling the handle to drag the head down your cheek. When the handle's dropped roughly 30° from the initial perpendicular (depending on the razor you're using), the blade will make contact with the whiskers and begin to cut stubble as you pull the razor.

That's the angle (more or less). The idea is that the edge of the blade is *cutting through* the whiskers, *not scraping over* them. If the room is quiet, you can hear the sound of the razor cutting through the whiskers. Think of the blade as being almost parallel to the skin, cutting the stubble at almost a right angle.

In the left photo, the razor is held at too shallow an angle, and the blade is not cutting. In the center photo, the blade (bent over the hump of the platform) is close to parallel to the skin and is cutting through stubble. In the right photo,

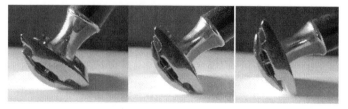

the handle is too low, so the blade is at too steep an angle and is scraping across the skin, producing razor burn.

Another image: think of the razor as a chain saw and the stubble as young saplings. You don't want to dig the chain saw into the ground (your skin), and you want it to cut through the saplings (stubble) more or less at right angles and close to the ground (skin). Another: think of the blade as gliding over a thin layer of lather like a toboggan over snow.

As the skin on your face curves this way and that—over the jawline, around the chin, and so on—you continually adjust the razor's angle by moving the handle to keep the blade almost parallel to the skin being shaved.

Using short strokes enables you to focus on blade angle (and pressure) for the entire stroke—and for a short stroke the angle is likely to be constant. Try locking fingers and wrist, using your arm to move the razor: this makes it easier to maintain a constant angle.

The correct cutting angle is different for different razors, and you determine the correct angle through feel and the sound the blade makes as you shave. Don't over-rely on feel: a double-edged blade is sharp enough so that you don't always feel the damage. Keep a close watch, and listen to the blade.

When I use my Gillette Super Speed, it's held flatter to the face than the Merkur Futur, for example. And with the Schick Injector and the Gem G-Bar, the cutting angle is when the razor's head is flat against the skin. You'll have to experiment to find the right cutting angle for each of your razors. As a rule of thumb, hold the razor so that the edge of the cap, which lies just behind the cutting edge of the blade, stays in contact with the skin. Don't pay attention to the guard; the correct angle can be found by keeping the edge of the cap and blade touching the skin. Think of the blade as sliding along over a layer of lather, not quite touching the skin.

One shaver has pointed out[151] that the correct angle is extremely important. Use as little pressure as you like, but if the angle is too steep, the blade will dig in and cut. He said that none of the instructions on the Internet **emphasize** this point sufficiently.

I had a tiny travel razor[152] with no handle: you hold it by the head. On shaving with it, I discovered that the tactile feedback from holding the head told me immediately if I stopped cutting and started scraping. One guy tried a similar approach[153] with a regular razor and found it helpful for getting the right feel.

So: hold the razor by the handle tip to feel the proper pressure, and hold it by the head to feel the proper angle. (These grips are for instructional purposes only—in your normal, day-to-day shave you don't use either of these.)

Proper technique consists of using light pressure and maintaining the correct blade angle over your entire beard area, including the neck.

In summary: Don't focus your attention on the razor's guard—forget about it. A novice who focuses his attention on the guard will generally get too steep a blade angle, thus scraping his face and producing razor burn. The guard is there if it's needed, so you don't have to think about it.

Put your attention instead on the edge of the cap, where the blade is exposed. Keep the cap's edge on your skin, and the angle will take care of itself. If you put the very top of the cap on your skin, the handle sticks out at right angles and the blade's edge is above the skin. Lower the handle until the blade touches the skin. Then the edge of the cap (just behind the blade's cutting edge) will be touching the skin, but make sure it's not *pressing* the skin—that is, it should be in contact with the skin, but no more than that. (Imagine you're shaving a balloon.) This combination—edge of cap touching the skin (for angle) but not enough to press into the skin (for pressure)—will minimize cuts and eliminate razor burn. If the cap is not in contact with the skin at all, with the razor riding on the guard, the angle is too steep and razor burn is likely.

Men who have already established shaving habits from using multiblade-cartridge razors will find that they automatically tend to hold the razor with the handle close to their face. With a DE razor, this puts the guard on the face and the blade at a steep angle, scraping the skin and causing razor burn.

The correct angle with a DE razor puts the handle far from the face (to keep the cap's edge on the skin), which feels strange to someone accustomed to a cartridge razor, and often his muscle-memory will lower the handle (which puts the guard firmly on the face, increasing blade angle and producing razor burn). The only way to avoid this is to pay careful attention. In much the same way, muscle memory of the pressure required by cartridge razors leads novices to use excess pressure with a DE razor—again the cure is careful conscious attention. Eventually, of course, new habits are established.

The grip

One shaver made a useful discovery regarding how to hold a razor, though (like many good discoveries) it sounds obvious once you're told: hold the razor at the point of balance.

He pointed out that both the Futur and the Vision have a definite waist, unlike most razor handles, and both are heavier than the typical razor. He wondered whether the waist was designed to show the center of balance and the right place for the grip.

For him (and me, as well), it works well: it's easier to control angle and pressure if you hold your razor at the point of balance.

When you grip the razor, your grip should be *light*, not tight—no more tightly than you would hold a sparrow, for example: tightly enough so that it cannot escape, but not so tightly as to harm it. (These are the same instructions given to beginning fencers on how to hold the foil: enough for control, not so much as to cause tension and tiredness.)

The sound

Make sure your bathroom is quiet: turn off the fan, turn off the radio, turn off any running water. When it's quiet, you can hear the sound of shaving. (The noise of running water is another reason that shaving in the shower is a bad idea.)

This is not some Zen idea (though the sound is certainly pleasant in a contemplative way). Rather, by listening to the sound made by your blade and razor as you shave, you can tell how the shave is going: the sound of scraping your face (bad) is unlike the crisp sound of each whisker being cut (good).

Some razors—notably the Progress, the Futur, and the Vision—seem to hold the blade so that the sound is amplified and you can hear even more clearly the little drama taking place under the lather where blade meets the stubble, but with any razor you can hear the sound of shaving if your bathroom is quiet. That auditory feedback is valuable: use it wisely.

Here we go

Recall the grain directions over your entire beard, referring if necessary to the diagram you made in Chapter Six. If you're in a situation in which you have to carry your shave kit to the bathroom and back (as in a dormitory), you can use a Rubbermaid or Tupperware container as the box: carry the kit to the bathroom, use the container while there to hold the water for your shave if you use the sink-full-of-water method (so you don't have to clean out the sink), then at the end of the shave, rinse out and dry the container, pack your kit back in, and return with it to your room.

Do your prep—and take enough time to do a thorough job and ensure the stubble is ready for the razor—pick up your razor, rinse the head under hot water (because cold metal against the cheek is unpleasant), chant, "Light pressure, correct blade angle," and set to work on the first pass.

The mirror sometimes gets covered with condensation. To prevent this, spread some lather on the mirror, then wipe it clean. Or use a little liquid soap on the mirrors, spread it around with a paper towel or toilet paper, then wipe it clean. This prevents condensation easily, and the lather's right at hand.

First pass: With the grain

Your first pass is *with* the grain (WTG). The second pass will be *across* the grain (XTG), either directly across or across at a slant. Those who do XTG at a slant usually do a second XTG pass on the opposite slant. Only the final pass will be against the grain (ATG), and in the beginning you should skip this pass, introducing it gradually as described below.

Again: use short strokes, light pressure, and keep the correct blade angle for the entire stroke, Keep your attention focused, and your technique (and results) will improve from shave to shave as you gain experience.

Of course, as with all advice regarding shaving: try short strokes, and see how they work for you. But the long, sweeping strokes possible with a pivot-headed cartridge razor will not work so well with the non-pivoting safety razor.

Stretching the skin where you're shaving can help lift the whiskers, and taut skin is less likely to be cut. Stretch the skin against the grain to raise the stubble for cutting, or you can contort your face by grimacing or puffing out your cheeks. Experiment with different techniques to find those that work for you. Brush your wet fingers over an alum block (discussed later) to grip the skin, or use a damp washcloth in your stretching hand. (Generally, for the skin around your mouth, grimacing is enough.) Shave away from the hand that's stretching the skin. The skin under the chin is easily stretched by lifting your chin.

The upper lip is tricky because the nose is not removable. Fortunately, though, the nose is flexible, so with your free hand, you can push or pull the nose to one side or upward to give your razor more room to work. You also can shave under the nose—the philtrum area—by coming down from either side at a slant.

To stretch the skin of my upper lip, I simply draw my lip down over my teeth. Some push their tongue between the front teeth and the lip.

The Adam's apple presents a problem for some guys. One technique is to pull the skin to the side, where it's flatter: simply grip some neck skin between your fingers and pull to the side. Another trick is to swallow and hold it—that flattens the Adam's apple long enough for you to shave it. As you shave your neck, pay especially close attention to blade angle and to pressure and to the grain. The neck presents a tricky area in shaving.

Another spot difficult for many is the jawline. On some guys, the jawline is a rather sharp curve, easily navigated with a multiblade cartridge because of its pivoting head, but with the safety razor you yourself must manage the angle changes to keep the blade almost parallel to the skin being shaved: a DE razor is a "manual transmission," not "automatic." When the skin curves, you must move the handle to keep the head properly aligned. At the jawline this generally means lots of handle movement. Short strokes help—in a short distance, the skin direction is less apt to change drastically. You also can use the same trick here as for the Adam's apple: pull the skin on the curve to a flatter place and shave it there.

The safety razor has two sides, and in shaving you flip back and forth, using both edges of the double-edged blade. After the razor's head has accumulated lather from a few strokes, flip it to the "clean side" until that, too, is filled with lather, then rinse and repeat. After each rinse, give it a good shake to remove water before resuming the shave.

When you rinse your face after the first pass, you'll feel stubble. That's fine. You will be doing another pass, and each pass further reduces the stubble, with the end result a smooth face. Do **not** increase pressure in an attempt to remove stubble faster: you'll remove a thin layer of skin along with the stubble.

Second pass: Across the grain

Once you complete the first (WTG) pass, rinse your face and re-lather. (Lather is always applied to a wet beard.) The second pass is across the grain (XTG), and this further reduces the stubble. The XTG pass is particularly useful for reducing the tough stubble on the upper lip. In fact, I go *both* directions XTG on my upper lip and on my chin. The stubble there is particularly tough, and by minimizing it as much as possible, the against-the-grain pass becomes much easier. I don't relather between those two XTG passes in those areas, but try it with relathering and without relathering to see which works best for you. Always experiment: you will then develop a technique that matches your unique shaving situation.

Again: light pressure, correct blade angle, and short strokes, with your attention focused on what you're doing.

Rinse, and—when you first start shaving with a safety razor—that's it. If you want further stubble reduction, you can re-lather after rinsing and do another XTG pass, going the other direction, but when you first start using the safety razor, *don't shave ATG*, for two reasons. First, until you master blade angle and pressure, ATG is likely to cause cuts and/or skin irritation. Second, in the ATG pass, you hold the razor upside down, and more practice and concentration are needed to keep pressure and angle correct in that maneuver.

Third pass: Against the grain

When you are ready to shave ATG: rinse your beard before that pass and feel the stubble. The stubble should be almost gone—if it's not, do an XTG pass the other way. Before the ATG pass, you want the stubble truly minimized. If you are prone to getting razor bumps in some areas, do not do an ATG pass in those areas.

When you first start doing ATG, re-lather your wet beard after the XTG and do ATG *only on your cheeks and sideburn area*. That's the easiest area and will give you good practice without getting into the difficult curves and challenges of chin, jaw, neck, etc. After a few shaves, when you're happy with ATG on your cheeks and are comfortable with the ATG razor position, do your chin as well, then your upper lip, and finally your neck and under the jaw. Remember to keep a correct blade angle for the skin you're shaving, as the skin curves this way and that, and remember to use light pressure. Again: short strokes allow you to focus on angle and pressure for the entire stroke.

Enchante Online has a useful diagram[154] on the direction of the cutting strokes (assuming "normal" beard grain). I got a fine shave when I used some of this pattern, modifying it as dictated by my own beard. (For example, I use XTG on my upper lip.)

For a thorough shave, try a **four-pass shave**: WTG, XTG on a slant, XTG on the other slant, and ATG. You can modify the basic four-pass method[155] to suit the lineaments of your own face. The benefit of this method is how completely it reduces the stubble so the final, ATG pass is quite comfortable.

Going for a clean, close shave in one pass results in too much pressure, a guarantee of razor burn and cuts—progressive reduction through multiple passes is the key.

I usually do a **three-pass shave**: WTG, XTG (ear-toward-nose), and ATG. As I mentioned, one small patch at the heel of my right jaw grows horizontally toward my chin, so with the usual three passes that particular patch never got an against-the-grain pass. So now my three passes include one little backward horizontal pass over that spot. And my ATG pass on my right cheek, near the mouth, tilts to match the grain pattern of my beard there.

For me, as for most men, the beard on chin and upper lip is particularly tough, which is why I do XTG both directions in those places—again, to reduce the stubble as much as possible before the ATG pass.

Do not do an ATG pass in areas in which you get in-growns.

The polishing pass [optional]

Once you're doing the ATG pass, you can finish the shave with a polishing pass to remove the last traces of roughness. Do *not* do a polishing pass where you get razor bumps—in such areas you want to avoid shaving closely at all. Three ways of doing the polishing pass are a water pass, an oil pass, and a pre-shave pass.

The water pass

The water pass works well as a natural extension of the final (ATG) pass, especially if during the ATG pass you're using your non-razor hand to stretch the skin. After finishing that ATG pass, rub your face with your wet left hand (assuming you're right handed—with the non-razor hand, in any case).

When you find a rough patch, use "blade buffing" to remove it: keeping the proper angle and light pressure while doing extremely short ATG strokes, on the order of 1/4" or less, not lifting the blade as you move it back and forth. One shaver described the motion as if you were trying to scribble in a small section of your beard with a pencil. Blade buffing is one of the advanced shaving techniques[156] that experienced shavers use in the final passes.

Another advanced shaving technique, the J-hook, often works well on the neck. One shaver reported that he used the J-hook (a final-pass technique, remember), both clockwise and counterclockwise, and got a much smoother result with no irritation. Again: experiment.

The water from your hand as you feel for roughness, together with the residue of the lather, provides lubricity, and because you are shaving with only water and whatever tiny bit of lather remains, the shave is naturally close enough to remove even very short stubble.

If too little lather residue is left on your face, squeeze the bristles of your shaving brush with the fingers of your left hand. Then as you feel for rough spots, you will apply a bit of lather to your face. The left hand does double duty, both feeling for roughness and stretching the skin as needed, and if it's already been doing that through the third pass, the transition to the water pass is seamless.

Although the water pass works, I usually prefer the oil pass, which I find effective and pleasant, during and after.

The oil pass

In Method shaving (described at the end of the chapter), the final pass is a "touch-up" using their Hydrolast Cutting Balm, a combination of oils and essential oils. The Cutting Balm pass works extremely well, so it's a natural step to try other oils.

The idea is this: after you finish your regular shave—for me, a three-pass shave (with, across, and finally against the grain, lathering before each pass)—rinse well, apply a few drops of oil to the palm of your left hand (assuming you hold your razor in your right), rub it over your **wet** beard, and then do a "polishing" pass, feeling with your left hand for rough spots, then buffing those with the razor against the grain.

Rinse, dry your face with a towel (which removes most of the oil, with the oil remaining acting as a skin conditioner), and apply aftershave of choice. If you want to use an alum block as described below, use it after that final rinse.

My current "complete" shave, though step 5 is often omitted:
1. Wash beard with MR GLO or Whole Foods 365 glycerin soap.
2. Rinse. Lather. Pass 1 (WTG)
3. Rinse. Lather. Pass 2 (XTG), both directions on chin and lips.
4. Rinse. Lather. Pass 3 (ATG)
5. Rinse. Either: Glide alum bar over face and let sit a moment; or:
   Rub 2-5 drops oil on wet beard area. Do polishing pass.

6. Rinse. Towel dry.

7. Apply aftershave.

Commercial shave oils

I had excellent results with the oil pass, so I experimented with different oils. I tried a variety of commercial oils, almost all of which identify themselves as "pre-shave" oil. I, however, use them only for the oil pass.

Art of Shaving shave oil is generally judged by those who have tried it as being much too thick and gummy and altogether unsatisfactory, so I skipped that one. True to YMMV, however, some shavers say they do like this oil.

Hydrolast Cutting Balm[157] is but one component of the Method shave system (described below), but it can be used on its own. It's a "proprietary blend of vegetal oils, proprietary blend of essential oils." This was the origin of the oil pass idea, thanks to Charles Roberts of Method shave fame. It's very nice: light fragrance, light oil, and does a great job.

Total Shaving Solution[158]: This oil seemed *very* mentholated, so it should appeal to menthol fans. Very slick, light, and does the job.

All Natural Shaving Oil[159]: Often called Pacific Shaving Oil since it's made by Pacific Shaving Company. This oil seems to have some emulsifiers which make it mix with the water, but it still provides an excellent surface for the oil pass. Though it lists menthol among the ingredients, the menthol is subdued.

King of Shaves Kinexium ST Shaving Oil[160]: This one easily wins the prize for packaging: a little flip-top lid that hinges open, a press button that produces exactly the right amount. It does a good job, but the fragrance is somewhat off-putting—to me, it's like machine-oil.

Gessato Pre-Shave Oil[161]: This oil is light and clear and has no discernible fragrance, a benefit. Does a very nice job, but is somewhat pricey.

Oils from the supermarket

You can also use oils you find at the supermarket. All of those listed below are non-comedogenic oils[162]—that is, oils that have a very low probability of clogging pores. However, some people are more apt to get clogged pores than others, so you should (as always) be guided by your own experience.

All of the oils listed below have well established histories of cosmetic use and don't go rancid (as would, say, flaxseed oil). They all are listed as being good for the skin. And except for Jojoba oil, they all are good oils for cooking or salads, so they certainly don't have to be reserved exclusively for shaving—the oil pass requires very little oil, in any event, so you'll have plenty of oil left over for other uses. I recommend against using mineral oil (or products based on mineral oil) on your skin; mineral oil is a petroleum derivative.

- Almond oil
- Avocado oil
- Grapeseed oil (good used just by itself)
- Jojoba oil (good used just by itself)
- Macadamia nut oil
- Olive oil (good used just by itself)

Leisureguy's Last-Pass Shaving Oil: I used a combination of the above to make an oil-pass mix. Alter the formula as you want—there's really nothing special about the mix I made, though it works for me. It is, however, thicker than the commercial oils listed above.

2 parts Almond oil
2 parts Avocado oil
2 parts Olive oil
1 part Grapeseed oil
1 part Macadamia nut oil
1-2 drops essential oil(s) (for fragrance)—as much as you want

It's important to add only *one* (1) drop of the essential oil and then try the mix—you can always add another drop, but removing a drop is difficult.

Useful equivalences for making small batches: 2 Tablespoons = 1 fluid ounce, and 3 teaspoons = 1 Tablespoon. Knowing this, you can readily figure out how many ounces you'll make if you use regular measuring spoons: for example, if 1 part = 1 tsp, the above formula will result in 1 1/3 fl oz, which is plenty for a batch—that much will last you a long time. If 1 part = 1 Tbsp, the result is 4 fl oz (that is, 1/2 cup), which is a *lot* of oil—enough to share with friends.

You can readily find plastic dispensers in natural[163] or cobalt blue[164] or other colors. The "treatment pump" top (available in white or black) works just right to dispense a drop or two per push: exactly the right top for this application. If you buy one of the commercial oils in a larger container, you might want to decant an ounce into one of these little bottles with the treatment pump to use in travel (or at home).

Baby massage oils generally have good ingredients—babies frequently put their fingers and toes into their mouths, so these oils are made with harmless edible ingredients—but always read the label carefully. A search on "baby massage oil" will find a wide selection for your consideration. Look for organic natural ingredients and try one of those.

You can let the shave oil container sit in warm water while you shave so that it's comfortably warm when it's applied after the final pass.

Pre-shaves for a polishing pass

The commercial oils used for the polishing pass are mostly identified as "pre-shave" oils. And, as you might suspect, you can use other pre-shaves for a polishing pass: Proraso Pre- and Post-Shave Cream, PREP, or Crema 3P.

A different razor for each pass

Bruce Everiss came up with the idea, mentioned earlier, of using the most appropriate razor for each pass: the three-razor method (assuming that, like most shavers, your typical shave consists of three passes). For example:

> First pass (WTG): Bulk removal: Slant Bar
> Second pass (XTG): Smoothing the face: Edwin Jagger DE8x
> Third pass (ATG): Polishing pass: A Super Speed or Tech

Obviously, the blade also can be chosen with an eye to the nature of the particular task each pass must perform (and, as noted earlier, the same brand of blade can perform differently in different razors).

The three-razor technique is much simpler than it may at first seem. Most shavers who have multiple razors keep several razors in rotation, already loaded with blades and ready for use. The shaver simply takes the appropriate razor, shaves one pass with it, rinses it, places it back on the shelf or in the rack, and picks up the appropriate razor for the next pass.

With the razors loaded and ready to go, changing razors between passes is totally trivial, especially since you already rinse the razor between passes. The only added task is to set down the razor used in the previous pass and pick up the razor for the next pass.

Another situation in which a change in razor might be useful is described in the Slant Bar section: when you have a spot (at the corner of your mouth, for example) that feels rough after shaving, even though you took care to shave against the grain at that spot and could feel no stubble remaining when you check. Yet later in the day the little rough patch still is present.

Very thin whiskers, when cut short and fully wetted, are imperceptible to the touch (because then they are so soft), and a regular razor, pushing the blade straight at them, simply pushes them over without cutting them (because then they're so flexible that they bend readily under the pressure of the cutting edge, lacking the rigidity to stand upright and be cut).

If you have stubble of this sort, use a Slant Bar for the polishing pass in that area. The slanted blade, acting as a guillotine rather than simply pushing straight at the stubble will cut even soft, thin whiskers before they can bend aside. Obviously, of course, you can simply use the Slant Bar for the entire shave.

Choosing the appropriate razor for the task/pass at hand is worth a try, assuming you have a collection of razors with different shaving characteristics.

Method Shaving

Charles Roberts of EnchanteOnline.com developed a method of shaving that some shavers really like. He uses some special supplies, and recommends the Merkur HD razor and a sharp blade. The special supplies consist of:

- The Shavemaster brush—or any large, fan-type brush
- An olive-oil soap, originally "The Cube" but now rounds
- A shaving paste used with the soap to produce the lather
- "Activator," a product to help in lather production
- Cutting balm, discussed above
- Skin tonic and conditioner

A good introduction to Method shaving is provided by three videos made by Mantic59[165]. The supplies listed are available online[166].

My own experience with Method shaving was generally positive. Because the lather depends on the proportions of soap, shaving paste, and Activator, it tends to vary somewhat from session to session, at least until you become skilled in creating the mix. The Shavemaster brush is large and works well to generate a lather from soap—if you have large hands, you're likely to be particularly appreciative of the brush. But, as noted, you can use any large brush.

Although I use Method shaving only occasionally, I do enjoy having it in my repertoire. If you're experimentally minded, give it a go.

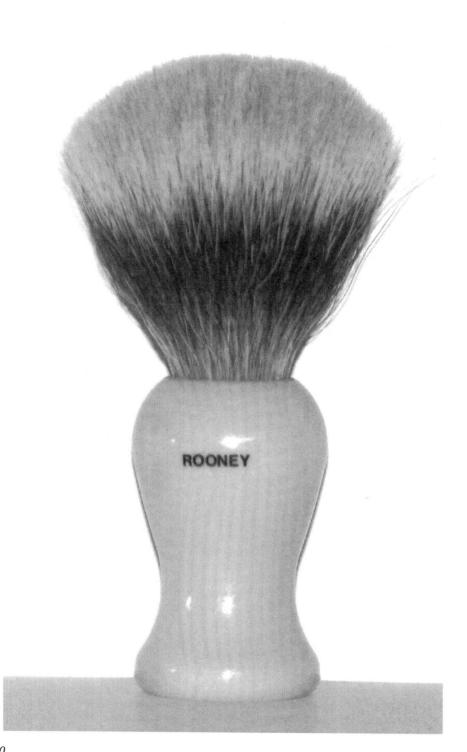

ELEVEN

The post-shave routine

AFTER you finish your shave, rinse your razor in hot water and leave it out to dry. If you're using a carbon-steel blade, or if you have hard water, or if you have acne or get razor bumps, rinse the razor head in high-percentage rubbing alcohol (91% or higher), which drives out the water and then immediately evaporates, leaving the blade dry and without hard-water deposits.

There's no need to remove the blade or even to loosen the razor's grip on the blade. In general, it's a good idea to minimize handling the blade: remove it only to discard it. Lay the razor on its side; a razor stand is not necessary.

Rinse out your brush—first with warm water until the lather's gone, then with cold water. Shake it well, dry it on a towel if you want, then stand it on its base in the open to dry. A brush stand is not necessary.

After you put the razor and brush away, rinse your face first with warm water and then with cold—quite refreshing.

The alum block

After the cold-water rinse and prior to using an aftershave, definitely try using an alum block. It's extraordinarily refreshing, but something that (like coffee) appeals primarily to adults: the sensation is a tingling and sometimes a slight stinging. It will stop weepers from bleeding, but that is not its purpose.

The alum block is an antiseptic and seems to be highly beneficial for those who suffer from acne or other skin problems. A common comment from a new wetshaver is that once an alum block becomes a regular post-shave routine, skin blemishes in the beard area simply stop occurring. And, of course, one gets good feedback on shaving technique: a better shave results in less sting.

One good-sized alum block should last for a year or two (unless you drop it on a hard floor). According to Shavex, which makes the alum blocks sold by Mama Bear: "The Alum Block (for shaving and deodorant purposes) is usually Potash Alum. Potash Alum doesn't sting so much as Ammonium Alum, but some companies do use Ammonium Alum as a shaving block."

Potassium Alum (another name for Potash Alum) is used in some deodorant crystal sticks, and for some reason these are often priced much less than alum blocks sold to shavers. Naturally Fresh makes a deodorant crystal of potassium alum with aloe vera. (Some deodorant crystals are made with Ammonium Alum, so be sure to check—though "mineral crystal" may be the only information.) The Wikipedia article on Alum[167] provides more information.

RazoRock is a potassium alum block in stick form, nicely packaged in a travel container and specifically intended and designed for aftershave use.

Whether you use the block daily, weekly, or not at all will depend on how your skin reacts. Most find that an alum block works fine and with no problems, some must use it sparingly, and a few must avoid it altogether. If the alum block causes your skin to redden, similar to razor burn, you may be one of the unlucky few. Some have reported that the alum block seems to interact with Nivea aftershave balm to produce irritation.

Glide the alum block over your freshly shaved part of your face while your face is still wet from the cold-water rinse. (No need to wet the block: the water remaining on your face is ample.) Do not press—*glide* the block, don't push it. The action is non-abrasive: the block simply slides lightly over your wet, freshly shaved face. Then let the block air-dry. I use a wooden ladder-style soap rack: it's best not to let wet alum rest on or near metal because it's reactive and wet alum will in time corrode metal. Store it dry.

In hot weather, try keeping the alum bar in the freezer, bringing it out just before you shave: the frigid bar gliding over your wet, freshly shaved skin is a wonderful sensation.

I have read instances in which some have inexplicably attempted to use a styptic pencil as though it were an alum block, rubbing the side of the pencil on the face. This is misguided. The styptic pencil is not the same substance; it's usually aluminum sulfate anhydrous or titanium dioxide. Get a real alum block.

The alum block has multiple uses. One woman notes[168] that the alum block seems to take care of pimples—she just washes her face with water and then glides the alum block over her wet face and follows that with Thayers Rose Petal Witch Hazel. The result: no pimples, and no residual powder from the alum block. (She says it also stops the stinging on bug bites.) Also, those with skin blemishes may want to use the alum block even on non-shave days.

And as noted earlier an alum block helps to get a secure grip (on wet, soapy skin or the razor): just run your wet fingertips over the block.

When I use an alum block, I let my alum-blocked face drip while I rinse my brush—first with hot water, then with cold—then shake it well and put it out dry. (My brushes dry standing in the open on their base.) Then I police the sink area, putting things away and using a sponge to wipe up splashed water.

I then rinse the alum from my face (it's important to rinse after using an alum block: otherwise the alum dries the skin), dry my face, and apply an aftershave. And that's it: the shave is complete.

Some see that aluminum in the chemical formula and become concerned. First, note that sodium and chlorine are both present in sodium chloride (table salt), and though both individually are dangerous, the compound is not only safe but in fact essential for health. Second, aluminum is simply not the danger that it was once thought to be[169].

Styptics

The alum block is primarily a skin treatment, as noted above, though it will stop bleeding from weepers. But to staunch a nick, a styptic is much better than an alum block (though powdered alum does make a good and inexpensive styptic: dip your fingertip in the powder and press onto nick to stop bleeding).

If I have a nick or cut (nowadays rare), I use My Nik Is Sealed[170], a liquid styptic in a roll-on applicator. It works like a charm, *much* better than a styptic pencil, and it doesn't leave white deposits on your face as a styptic pencil does. I find that this product has very little sting—for me: individuals vary in their response to styptic. Other forms of liquid styptic are Pacific Shaving Company's Nick Stick (though it doesn't work quite as well as MNIS) and Proraso's Styptic Gel[171]. The least expensive liquid styptic, which you can apply by putting a drop or two on a Q-Tip and then daubing the cut, is KDS-Lab Liquid Styptic[172]. In my own experience My Nik Is Sealed works best of the lot.

Aftershaves

The shaving products previously mentioned—shaving brushes, shaving soaps and creams, double-edged blades, safety razors—have a somewhat limited market: men who have discovered the benefits of traditional wetshaving. The marketing dollars that create infinite new variations, and the advertising dollars that work to convince ~~gullible victims~~ potential customers of the wondrous benefits of the latest variation—even if it's only changing the color of the plastic in the razor's handle—are markedly absent for traditional wetshaving.

But now we reach aftershaves—products sold to *every* shaver—so here you will find incredible variety. Badger & Blade has a lengthy review[173] that covers just some of the products available, sorted by skin type (dry, normal, combination, and oily). And Mantic59 devotes one of his excellent shaving videos specifically to aftershaves[174].

Generally speaking, you can choose among an aftershave (bracing) or a balm (soothing) or a gel (moisturizing). Some shavers have found that their skin (particularly in bad weather) simply can't take alcohol-based aftershaves.[175]

Many kinds of gel are available: Gillette gels, and also Anherb from India, Tabiano from Italy, and Arko from Turkey, and Taylor of Old Bond Street from the UK. For razor burn, aloe vera gel works well (as does plain jojoba oil).

Thayers Witch Hazel is available at drugstores and health food stores and comes in a variety of fragrances[176], none of which linger. (Thayers has a sampler pack[177] of their various witch hazels.) There's also a Thayers Witch Hazel Aftershave[178], a bit more bracing and an excellent aftershave if you're traveling or if you're a night shaver: it has no fragrance. (It's a 4-oz. bottle, but you'll be checking your shaving things anyway: blades.) Some guys add a few drops of tea-tree oil to their witch-hazel to make an even more restorative aftershave—worth considering if you're fighting some skin conditions.

Dickerson's witch hazel is commonly available, but has what some consider an offensive odor. A little fragrance or drop of tea-tree oil helps.

Some aftershaves that I've tried and especially liked: Klar Seifen Klassik, TOBS Mr. Taylor's and Shave Shop and Sandalwood (though note that Sandalwood seems to trigger sensitivities fairly often), Dominica Bay Rum, Pashana, Trumper Spanish Leather, Trumper West Indian Extract of Limes (with a wonderfully intense fresh lime fragrance), and the various types of Floïd aftershave. Pinaud Clubman has a nice old-timey fragrance. Some continue to swear by Old Spice, Mennen Skin Bracer, Barbasol, or Aqua Velva, which can be found at your local drugstore. Some aftershaves are preparations specifically made to treat razor bumps. These are discussed in the next chapter.

The artisanal soap makers—Em's Shave Place, Honeybee Soaps, Mama Bear, QED, Saint Charles Shave, and others—also make aftershave lotions and balms that are well worth trying. I have a large collection of Saint Charles Shave aftershave splashes: excellent and quite different from commercial products. I highly recommend you try some samples of those. And Captain's Choice Bay Rum is a terrific bay rum aftershave—with no cloves.

Appleton Barber Supply offers a great variety of aftershaves, including many old-time favorites. Booster's aftershaves[179] from Canada are modestly priced and very nice—June Clover is a favorite.

If you want a balm as an aftershave treatment, look (at your drugstore, for example) for Neutrogena Razor Defense lotion, Triple Defense cream, or Nivea Aftershave Sensitive lotion. Experiment with applying those balms while your beard is still wet following the final rinse. Barclay Crocker offers a very nice aftershave balm. Aftershave balms by l'Occitane and Institut Karité include shea butter and work quite well for moisturizing your skin. A very nice balm is Shea Moisture Three-Butters Balm (avocado, mango, and shea butter).

Both Taylor of Old Bond Street's Luxury Herbal Aftershave Cream and the Geo. F. Trumper Skin Foods (Coral (rose), Sandalwood, or Lime) are quite good aftershave balms. Proraso's pre- and after-shave cream[180] works well as an aftershave balm. Some particularly good balms are Primalan (almond-oil based), Alt-Innsbruck (which also has a terrific splash), and Institut Karité 25% shea butter. Only a pea-sized amount is needed, so the bottle lasts a long time. When looking at prices, also look at the amount you get: all three of those last mentioned are around $30, but the first two are in 100ml bottles and the Institut Karité is in a 250ml bottle: two-and-a-half times as much for the same price.

A blog reader passed along his recipe for an aftershave balm. He makes only a small quantity at a time because it does not include a preservative.

1. Mix equal parts of witch hazel (he uses a high-quality witch hazel from a supplies shop) and Aloe Vera gel. Try 50 ml (1/4 cup) each. Mix with a mixer or blender to blend well.
2. Add a little glycerin (you can try with and without to see how you like the glycerin): 5-10 ml (1-2 tsp)
3. Add a little Lime essential oil (or Lavender or ...) for fragrance
4. Add a little water to thin it if you want. Or you can leave it as a gel and dip it from a tub with your fingers.

He says that it's as close to Castle Forbes Lime as you get without the price tag. He uses an eggbeater to mix the ingredients—though a whisk would probably work as well. The ingredients must be mixed well. It's the gel in the Aloe Vera gel that makes it balm-like—water is added just to thin it if you want to keep it in a bottle instead of a tub. Only a little is required. Aloe Vera has proved to be very good for razor burn.

In adding the essential oil, add just one drop, shake, let sit, and see how you like it. If not enough, add one more drop—it's very easy to add too much, so caution is advised. You might want to experiment using one of the Thayers witch-hazel-and-aloe-vera toners (no alcohol) or astringents (a little alcohol) as the base for your homemade aftershave.

If you get into making your own aftershaves or fragrances, take a look at CreatingPerfume.com, which offers things like perfumer's alcohol.

Aftershaves and colognes in retail stores have a high markup. Look at on-line discounters such as FragranceNet.com or check for bargains on eBay.

The particular fragrance of the aftershave is important because, unlike the fragrance of the pre-shave soap and the shaving soap or shaving cream, the aftershave fragrance will linger for a while. I don't attempt to describe the fragrances of the various aftershaves because my nose is illiterate, as it were. (A man with a highly educated nose is profiled in Chandler Burr's informative and fascinating book *The Emperor of Scent: A Story of Perfume, Obsession, and the Last Mystery of the Senses*[181]—highly recommended.) As observed earlier, anyone's nose will over time become habituated to a fragrance, which can lead to using too much fragrance (because it becomes harder to smell as you get used to it). Be careful of this if you use the same fragrance daily.

Some information on the relative fragrance strength of various dilutions of perfumes can be useful. From Wikipedia[182]:

> Perfume types reflect the concentration of aromatic compounds in a solvent, which in fine fragrance is typically ethanol or a mix of water and ethanol. Various sources differ considerably in the definitions of perfume types. The concentration by percent/volume of perfume oil is as follows:
>
> - Perfume extract (Extrait): 15-40% (IFRA: typical 20%) aromatic compounds
> - Eau de Parfum (EdP), Parfum de Toilette (PdT): 10-20% (typical ~15%) aromatic compounds. Sometimes listed as "eau de perfume" or "millésime".
> - Eau de Toilette (EdT): 5-15% (typical ~10%) aromatic compounds
> - Eau de Cologne (EdC): Chypre citrus type perfumes with 3-8% (typical ~5%) aromatic compounds
> - Splash and Aftershave: 1-3% aromatic compounds
>
> Perfume oils are often diluted with a solvent, though this is not always the case, and its necessity is disputed. By far the most common solvent for perfume oil dilution is ethanol or a mixture of ethanol and water. Perfume oil can also be diluted by means of neutral-smelling oils such as fractionated coconut oil, or liquid waxes such as jojoba oil.

If you discover that an aftershave you like (such as New York, by Parfums de Nicolaï) is no longer available but the corresponding Eau de Toilette is still on offer (and New York EDT is available), you could buy that and dilute it with a little water and/or alcohol to make an aftershave (or simply use a very small amount, perhaps while your face is still wet after the final rinse).

TWELVE

Skin problems

SOME shavers suffer specific skin problems: acne, razor bumps, and/or ingrown whiskers. Weather can trigger other skin issues—for example, shavers in cold climates know well what winter's cold dry air (and the hot dry air inside buildings) does to their skin, and shavers with curly beards may find that they get more ingrowns in humid weather.

This chapter addresses those problems, but only up to a point. Never assume that medical advice from a layperson is accurate. Dermatologists go to school for years because there's much to know, and they do much continuing study because new treatments and drugs regularly appear. What you learn in this section is not the final answer and may not even apply to your situation.

What I will explain are some suggestions from men who have tried various regimens and who describe what worked for them. It may or may not work for you because your skin, your general condition, your environment, and/or your problem may not correspond to their situation and their remedies. The same holds true for products mentioned: they work for some, but that doesn't mean that they will necessarily work for you: YMMV, as you recall.

For any of these conditions, however, shaving with a multiblade cartridge is a bad idea, even though multiblade cartridges are highly recommended by companies that make and sell them. But the tug-and-cut action of multiblade cartridges and the pressure exerted to make them work irritate the skin (bad for acne) and tugs out the whisker before cutting it (bad for razor bumps and ingrown whiskers). Single-blade shaving—either with a safety razor using a single- or double-edged blade, or with a straight razor—is much kinder to your skin once you have learned proper shaving preparation and techniques.

Acne

Acne is a skin problem that results from different causes, typically one (or a combination) of the following conditions:

- Excess sebum (an oily substance produced by certain cells)
- Rapid production of bacteria (which can live on the sebum)
- Skin cells shedding too quickly
- Inflammation resulting from the above

Acne can be mild[183], moderate[184], or severe[185] (endnotes are links to photos of the conditions). Mild acne can be treated at home, but moderate or severe acne is best treated with the care of a dermatologist. To see improvement once treatment begins may take as long as 4-8 weeks.

Note that your dermatologist may not be well-informed about shaving options and might, for example, recommend a multi-blade cartridge, even though that type of razor is strongly contraindicated.

Treatment of mild acne focuses on three things:

1. Avoiding skin irritation—avoid harsh scrubs, aggressive cleaning, rough brushes, strong soaps, and shaving with multiblade cartridges.
2. Keeping skin clean by gentle washing with a mild soap.
3. Applying preparations designed to treat acne.

Over-the-counter acne creams often contain benzoyl peroxide or salicylic acid. Benzoyl peroxide kills the bacteria that cause acne. Its principal side effect is excessive dryness of the skin, so don't use more than directed. Benzoyl peroxide also can bleach hair, sheets, towels, and clothing: be careful.

Salicylic acid helps correct abnormal skin shedding and helps unclog pores, but has no effect on sebum production or bacteria. Salicylic acid may be irritating to your skin, so you may not be able to use it—the general rule is always to avoid skin irritation.

Sulfur-based compounds work well for some (although there's some research[186] that shows that acne returns with increased severity after using sulfur-based compounds). In addition to over-the-counter treatments, prescription medicines are available through your doctor or dermatologist.

There's more information at AcneNet[187], and Acne.org[188] describes a good regimen. In terms of shaving, that regimen requires some extension.

1. When you wash your face, do it gently, using only your hands and a mild soap or cleanser. Do not use a washcloth or scrubber. Cetaphil cleanser is recommended by many dermatologists.
2. Use a fresh towel for each shave. You can buy thin, 100% lint-free cotton barber towels (aka bar towels) for about $11/dozen. Towels are microbe incubators, so this is a good step to take.

3. Use a fresh pillowcase each night. You can buy inexpensive pillowcases from hotel supply vendors.
4. Use a mild, unscented shaving soap or shaving cream, and a soft shaving brush rather than a "scrubby" one. Silvertip badger shaving brushes, for example, are quite soft and gentle, yet not floppy.
5. Swish the head of the razor in high-proof rubbing alcohol before and after each shave. Use a squat wide-mouth jar that formerly held a food product; those lids open/close with one-quarter turn. (You have to keep the alcohol in a closed container or it evaporates quickly.)
6. Use very light pressure when shaving and maintain a good blade angle. If you cut a pimple, apply a topical antiseptic to the cut.
7. You may find that you cannot use a shaving oil, even those having low comedogenicity[189]. If an oil makes the acne worse, give it up.
8. After the shave, try using an alum bar, which is a mild antiseptic. Glide the bar gently over your skin after the cold-water rinse, let it sit for a minute, then rinse and pat your skin dry with a towel. Do not rub. (You might add this step each time you wash your face.) Acne suffers frequently report that using the alum bar helps a lot.
9. Aftershaves or tonics containing alcohol may be too drying or irritating when used in combination with acne treatments. Try them to see whether they work for you or use a balm instead.
10. Some how found tea-tree oil has helped with their acne. Dr. Bronner makes a tea-tree soap, and you can try adding a couple of drops of tea-tree oil to witch hazel to use as an aftershave to see if it helps.
11. Wait until your skin is dry before applying any acne treatments.

More detailed instructions, including timings and amounts, are available at the site, which also offers products to help with the acne. Also note that Wicked_Edge has a useful reference post on acne and shaving[190].

The Mayo Clinic has a detailed series of articles[191] on acne, including information on causes and risk factors, when you should seek medical advice, and guidance on treatment, prevention, and self-care.

The book *Anticancer: A New Way of Life*[192] has this interesting passage:

When [Loren Cordain, PhD] was told that certain population groups whose way of life is very different from ours had no experience of acne (which is caused by an inflammation of the epidermis, among other mechanisms), he wanted to find out how this could occur... Cordain accompanied a team of dermatologists to examine the skin of 1,200 adolescents cut off from the rest of the world in the Kitavan Islands of New Guinea, and 130 Ache Indians living in isolation in Paraguay. In these two groups they found no trace whatsoever of acne. In their article in Archives of Dermatology, the researchers attributed their amazing discovery to the adolescents' nutrition. The diets of these contemporary sheltered groups resemble those of our distant ancestors: no refined sugar or white flour, thus no peaks of insulin or IGF in the blood.

In Australia, researchers convinced Western adolescents to try a diet restricting sugar and white flour for three months. In a few weeks, their insulin and IGF levels diminished. So did their acne.

Recently there have been important new findings on sugar's role[193].

Razor bumps and ingrown whiskers

Razor bumps are caused when hair cut close to the skin curls as it grows and either curls under the skin without emerging or curls into the skin next to where it emerged. Either event irritates the skin, causing inflammation. In some cases, infection follows, which causes a sore and drainage. Men who are African, Celtic, Mediterranean, Nordic, Semitic, or from other peoples who have naturally coarse or tightly curling hair often get 'razor bumps.'

The technical name is *Pseudofolliculitis Barbae*: "*pseudo*" (false) + "*follicle*" (hair) + "*itis*" (inflammation) + "*barbae*" (of the beard), often abbreviated as PFB. If the site becomes infected, "*pseudo*" no longer applies and the condition is called *Folliculitis Barbae* or "barber's rash." Photos of these conditions can be seen at the Dermatology Image Atlas[194].

Causes

The usual cause of PFB is shaving too closely. A multiblade cartridge, with its tug-and-cut action, is particularly bad: by tugging the whisker before it's cut, the cutting point is too close to the skin and can even be slightly beneath the skin's surface after the whisker pops back into place. But even a double-edged safety razor can deliver too close a shave, which leads to razor bumps. Electric razors, like multiblade cartridges, are particularly bad for men prone to PFB.

Shaving against the grain is a bad idea for the parts of your beard where you tend to get PFB, and stretching the skin as you shave there is equally bad. Both techniques are aimed at getting a closer shave, one source of the problem.

Another cause of PFB is irritation and damage to the skin from using a dull blade, or using a sharp blade with bad technique, or shaving after inadequate prep. All those should be avoided.

A common cause of infection is *Staphylococcus aureus* bacteria. The bacteria normally resides benignly in the nasal passages, but shaving can sometimes introduce it to hair follicles on the face. Once the hair follicle is infected, the result is redness, itching, and even small, pus-filled blisters. This is something that varies by individual—I've never had this problem, but some shavers are prone to such infection. Rinsing the razor in rubbing alcohol before and after the shave can help, as can using a fresh towel for every shave as described above in the section on acne.

Cures

If you now have razor bumps, stop shaving for a few days or a week—let the whiskers lengthen, and with a sterile needle release any whiskers caught in the skin or beneath the skin. If you have infected sites, apply an antibiotic and let the sites heal. Benzoyl peroxide can help, but apply it sparingly since it can be irritating. It's a good idea to see your doctor or a dermatologist, who can help with the diagnosis and prescribe appropriate medication.

Prevention

First is how you shave; second are products designed to prevent razor bumps.

Prep

Make sure that your preparation is thorough and excellent. You want the whiskers fully wetted so they will be more easily cut and less likely to be sharp at the cutting point. Shave after you shower. Use a softening conditioner on your beard in the shower. Use ample warm water to soften whiskers before shaving.

Wash your beard at the sink, using a good high-glycerin pre-shave soap such as Musgo Real Glyce Lime Oil soap or Whole Foods 365 brand glycerin soap. Rinse and, leaving your beard wet, apply a wet, hot towel or washcloth to your beard for 3-5 minutes. You can apply lather or Geo. F. Trumper's Coral Skin Food to your wet beard before the hot towel/washcloth if you find that this increases the wetting action of the towel. Place the hot wet towel over your lathered beard. Make sure this prep includes the shaving area of your neck as well as your face.

After removing the towel, rinse your beard with hot water, and then use a technique suggested by Themba[195] on the ShaveMyFace forum. He suggests using an Innomed Lice Comb[196]. (Moore Unique also makes a tool[197] for lifting the beard.) The comb is quite fine. As you comb against the grain, use firm but comfortable pressure and a shallow angle (as if shaving with the comb). This lifts the stubble and removes ingrowns and dead skin.

Then make a good (thick, wet, dense) lather from a good shaving soap or shaving cream, and brush it on your wet and combed beard against the grain.

Tools

Men who suffer from razor bumps say that the best razor to use is a straight razor. If you don't want to go that route, a single-edged razor—the Schick

Injector or the GEM G-Bar, both readily available on eBay—is, they say, just about as good. A double-edged razor also works well provided that you do not attempt to shave too closely. The Bump Fighter Razor[198] with its special Bump Guard blades is also recommended by some: it is specifically designed to prevent shaving too closely.

Use a new blade for each shave (if your blade is inexpensive) or else sterilize the blade before you begin each shave by rinsing it in a sterilizing solution. You can use rubbing alcohol (91% or higher) or a sterilizing product such as Ritual Razor Rinse (easily found with a Google search) or Barbicide[199].

Make sure the blade is sharp: discard blades before they become dull or at the first sign of tugging at the whiskers rather than cutting effortlessly.

Shaving

Consider shaving on alternate days, if that's possible for you. Shave bumpy areas last so the lather has more time to soften the stubble.

Don't stretch your skin while shaving places that get razor bumps. Stretching your skin while you shave increases the chance that a whisker will 'snap back' to below skin level when it's cut.

Shave with the grain and possibly across the grain, but never against the grain in areas prone to razor bumps—do not try for a totally smooth (close) shave in those areas. (You can shave against the grain in places where you never have razor bumps.)

If you cut a bump, apply an antibiotic to prevent infection. Use an alum bar after the shave, since it's a mild antiseptic. Just glide it over your skin after the cold-water rinse. Let it sit for minute—perhaps while you tidy up the shaving area—then rinse well with water, pat dry, and apply your shaving balm or aftershave or razor bump treatment. Rinse your beard area after the alum has had a chance to do its work. If using the alum doesn't seem to agree with your skin, stop using it. (Adverse reactions to an alum bar are rare, but given the variation among shavers, there's a possibility it can happen for some.)

Products

A number of over-the-counter products are specifically meant to prevent razor bumps. And through your doctor or dermatologist, you can get prescription medicines for the condition, such as eflornithine hydrochloride 13.9%, sold under the trade name Vaniqa. It's designed to remove facial hair for women, but it's apparently proven effective in controlling and treating razor bumps as well.

Following is a list of over-the-counter products. These—like most things in shaving—work for some, not for others. Posting questions in the shaving forums about any particular product will get you information from those who have used it. It would be a good idea to do a forum search before posting the question, though, since you may well find the product has been discussed.

Common products[200] (links at the endnote) that are used to combat razor bumps include the following:

Bump Fighter products (in particular the razor)
Bump Patrol
Dermagen Skin Revival System
Elicina Biological Treatment
Follique Treatment
High Time Bump Stopper Products
Moore Unique Skin Care
No Mo' Bumps Aftershave
Prince Reigns gel
Smart Shave Products
Tend Skin (you can make a version of Tend Skin at home[201])

Other skin issues

Eczema is a skin inflammation that has a number of causes, including (for some) some fragrances used in shampoo and conditioner.[202] If your skin suffers from dryness and recurring skin rashes characterized by redness, skin edema (swelling), itching and dryness, crusting, flaking, blistering, cracking, oozing, or bleeding, you may have one or another type of eczema, and you should see a dermatologist.

Winter's cold, windy weather and hot, dry air indoors can adversely affect a shaver's skin. Look for moisturizing products to help your skin: For shaving soaps, consider Mitchell Wool-Fat Shaving Soap or a shea-butter soap from Honeybee Soaps, Mama Bear, or Saint Charles Shave. Insitut Karité shaving soap contains 25% shea butter and produces an excellent lather.

Similarly, seek out moisturizing shaving creams. Saint Charles Shave offers a shea-butter shaving cream, or use Nancy Boy Shaving Cream—the Nancy Boy products in general are quite good for your skin. Institut Karité also makes shea butter shaving creams (20% and 25%).

For an aftershave, try Nancy Boy Body Moisturizer (heavier and cheaper than their face moisturizer and works quite well). Shea Moisture Three Butters Lotion works well; it uses avocado, mango, and shea butters. Cade aftershave balm by l'Occitane has a high shea-butter content. Primalan, an almond-oil based aftershave balm, and Alt-Innsbruck pre- and post-shave balm are both very good aftershave balms that come in 100ml containers; for about the same price,

Institut Karité has a 25% shea butter aftershave balm in a 250ml container. You need only a pea-sized amount of these balms.

Also you might try a tiny amount of The Shave Den's Pre-Shave Balm as a dry-air aftershave treatment because of its ingredients: Shea Butter, Lanolin, Jojoba Oil, Avocado Oil, Sweet Almond Oil, Vitamin E, and fragrance (sandalwood and oakmoss). I live in a very temperate climate and have little recent experience with dry air, summer or winter.

You can also use plain grapeseed oil or jojoba oil as a balm.

Em's Shave Place, Honeybee Soaps, Mama Bear, QED, Saint Charles Shave, and Barclay Crocker all offer soothing and moisturizing aftershave lotions and balms. You can email or call them to ask about the specific problem you're facing and get their informed opinions on the best approaches and products for you. In addition to any advice you get, pay attention to your own direct experience and see what in practice works best with your skin. Skin types vary widely, and it is not possible to give specific advice, so (once again) experimentation and close observation of results will be your best guide to what works for you.

THIRTEEN

Recommendations for a beginner

ON ShaveMyFace.com Rob_TN has an list of options for a beginner shaving kit[203] for someone on a limited budget (a student, for example). Bruce Everiss has selected a kit for a low-cost, high-luxury shave[204]. Whipped Dog offers a good and inexpensive beginner package to test whether DE shaving is for you[205].

Should you try any of these and find the experiment not work out for you, you can readily find buyers for the equipment and supplies in the Buying/Selling threads of shaving forums or reddit/r/shave_bazaar. Indeed, you might be able to get some of your equipment in the forums—along with advice (though sometimes inconsistent advice, though with sincere intention).

Hair conditioner instead of lather?

Some have found that they can use hair conditioner in place of shaving soap or shaving cream: they wash their beard at the sink with soap and water, then rinse it and apply the hair conditioner to the wet beard. After each pass, rinse the beard and apply hair conditioner again before the next pass.

This doesn't work for everyone, but if it works for you, you won't need a shaving brush, shaving soap, or shaving cream—so it may be worth a try. "Not working" means either some skin reaction to the hair conditioner or razor burn (red, burning skin) because the hair conditioner is not providing enough protection from the blade.

I did try it, and at first it seemed great. But then I had a difficult time seeing where I had shaved (the hair conditioner makes a thin and transparent layer), and I did get a fierce razor burn. So I returned to the traditional shaving cream or soap. I rate hair conditioner at best an emergency substitute for shaving soap or cream, and then for just one shave. Razor burn is unpleasant.

Women who shave their legs often use hair conditioner instead of lather, generally because they haven't tried a good lather and don't know its benefits.

Schick Injector as transitional razor

The Schick Injector (various models common on eBay, sometimes called the Schick Eversharp) offers a possible transitional razor for those accustomed to shaving with a cartridge razor. (Note that the pre-1960 Schick models are noticeably more aggressive than the later models, which still provide an excellent shave.) The Schick has somewhat the same feel as a cartridge razor, but uses a single-edged blade. The Schick (like the GEM G-Bar) is also a good razor for those who get razor bumps. On the whole, however, I strongly recommend starting with the traditional safety razor that uses a double-edged blade.

Leisureguy beginner shaving kit

A novice can split his transition from using canned foam and multiblade cartridges to traditional DE wetshaving into two steps, buying separately what is needed in each step. This has the budget advantage of breaking start-up costs into two purchases, perhaps a month apart.

Step 1 is *prep*: everything you need before you pick up the razor:

- **Pre-shave soap**: I like MR GLO, but Whole Foods 365 brand glycerin soap also works well; or try any other high-glycerin soap. No soap works well in hard water, so try distilled water if you're unsure of how soft your water is: that will show you if your water is hard.
- **Brush**: Whipped Dog Silvertip with resin handle (your choice). The 20mm or 22mm is the best all-round size (face or bowl lathering).
- **Shaving soap or shaving cream**: Try a variety of samples from Garry's Sample Shop and/or order samples from the artisanal soapmakers listed earlier. The best buy for excellent shaving cream is J.M. Fraser; for excellent shaving soap, Vitos Red Label Special.

In Step 1 your focus is on learning good prep: wash your beard with pre-shave soap at the sink using your hands and rinse partially with a splash. Then make a good lather and take your time working it into your beard. You may find the pre-shave soap lacks lubricity and/or it is difficult to get a good lather from shaving soap. If so, that may be due to hard water. Try the distilled water shave described previously. The difference can be astonishing.

Also determine the grain of your beard and start doing two passes, still using your multiblade-cartridge razor. Try using very light pressure. Do one pass with the grain and one pass across the grain, applying lather before each pass.

Step 2 is *shaving and aftershave*: everything for the rest of the shave:

- **Razor**: Although the Lord L6 or Feather Popular are inexpensive, they are (in effect) throwaway razors: you will eventually want to replace either. Moreover, the L6 is prone to breakage because of the flimsy aluminum handle. Those razors are also too light to use the pressure of the razor alone. On the other hand, they do allow you to try DE shaving at low cost. Still, I *strongly* recommend one of the Edwin Jagger DE8x series (or the Mühle equivalents): a lifetime razor with a reasonable weight. If your budget allows, one of the Weber razors (DLC or ARC) is a top-quality razor at a good price.
- **Blade sampler pack**: Buy a large pack with a good variety of blades. Initially try no more than four brands, then stick with the brand that seems to work best for two-three months so your technique can settle. At that point, explore the other brands. You may also want to include brands available in local stores, though those are costly.
- **Styptic**: I recommend My Nik Is Sealed or other liquid styptic. You will inevitably get a few nicks as you learn, and a liquid styptic staunches the bleeding more effectively than a styptic pencil.
- **Alum block**: The alum block as a post-shave skin treatment is pleasant and also seems effective against acne. It also offers a non-slip grip if you brush your wet fingers over it, on the one hand for your razor, on the other hand for gripping wet soapy skin to stretch it. You use a styptic only for nicks; you use an alum block after every shave.
- **Aftershave**: You can continue with your current aftershave, or experiment with a witch hazel (I recommend one of the Thayers line) or an aftershave splash or balm, depending on your tastes and needs.

You already know prep from Step 1, so now your focus is learn to use the razor. Read carefully the technique description and instructions that begin on page 121. By properly focusing your attention—and being careful to use light pressure—you can achieve a reasonably good result even with the first shave. Do just two passes: with the grain, rinse, relather, and across the grain. Your skill will improve from shave to shave if you pay attention and experiment carefully—trying different directions of cutting, for example: sometimes going at a slant (for under the nose and, for me, under the forward part of my jaw).

Recall the importance of keeping the edge of the cap in contact with the skin, which puts the razor's handle away from your face, and be careful to keep the pressure light. This will require much conscious attention at first, but eventually—and surprisingly soon—the adaptive unconscious learns the new practices so that intense conscious attention is no longer required.

Instead of the badger brush recommended above, you could go with a synthetic, horsehair, or boar brush. The safest choice is a synthetic: brushes of this type are totally reliable and consistent and a good choice for a beginner. Some like boar brushes because they are quite inexpensive. I like horsehair because it performs well.

Some shavers like to use a lathering bowl. A good choice would be a deep cereal bowl—approximately 5″ across, 3″ deep, with a hemispherical shape and a dark color so the lather is visible. I recommend trying without at first.

All of the above, Step 1 and Step 2, costs about the same as the price of 25-30 Fusion disposable cartridges.

If you tend to get razor bumps, consider the Bump Fighter razor[206], specifically designed to minimize razor bumps. Note that this razor is designed so that it will not give a close shave, even on the parts of your face where you never get razor bumps. With care, a regular DE razor works just as well.

I recommend that you get both a shaving cream and a shaving soap and practice with both from the start. For your first shaving soap, you might consider using a shave stick, since I find lather production is easiest using a shave stick (though men with sparse or soft beards will find a shave stick doesn't work). Shaving sticks are available in unscented versions. Palmolive, Lea, and Speick shave sticks all produce excellent lather at a low price, or get a shave stick from one of the artisanal soapmakers. Arko's shave stick (under $3) is also excellent.

If you want to try soap in a tub, let me recommend one the Honeybee Soaps or Mama Bear shaving soaps—those are made with shea butter and are quite nice to your skin. Strop Shoppe and Queen Charlotte soaps are also excellent. Or you might try a classic triple-milled shaving soap, such as Truefitt & Hill or D.R. Harris or Vintage Blades' own house brand. Dovo shave soap also is excellent. I suggest you use Garry's Sample Shop to try several soaps, and then buy tubs of those that work best for you.

For an aftershave, Bay Rum is a classic fragrance (and Captain's Choice is exceptional). Any of the various Thayers witch hazels work well. Or you might prefer a moisturizing balm after you shave; Neutrogena Razor Defense is one such and is available at your local drugstore.

For both equipment and supplies look in the Buying/Selling sections of the shaving forums and reddit's /r/shave_bazaar. You often can find bargains there. Post a "WTB" (Want To Buy) if you're looking for a specific item.

Your second razor

In time you will want a second razor (and—who knows?—perhaps a third and fourth). I have strongly recommend that your second razor be the Merkur Slant Bar. It should be a second razor because it requires a light touch and a sure hand, so it's best if you're experienced with a safety razor before using it.

The reason for this recommendation is the Slant Bar's unique cutting acting, which results in an extremely easy-cutting and smooth shave, an experience that most shavers enjoy: 70% of those who try a Slant Bar love it, and it doesn't work for only 7%.

A Slant Bar with a sharp blade is the ideal tool if you have a thick, wiry beard and sensitive skin. In my experience, the Slant will not give closer shaves than an excellent straight bar razor, but it's a different shave experience.

A recent poll on ShaveMyFace.com[207] indicated that a majority of those who had used both the Merkur HD and Slant Bar razors thought the Slant Bar was better, and only a small minority thought the HD was better. In all, 88% thought that the Slant Bar was better than or as good as the HD:

> If you've used both Slant Bar and HD, what do you find?
> Essentially no difference between them   30% [9]
> Slant Bar noticeably better than HD   58% [18]
> HD noticeably better than Slant Bar   13% [4] Total Votes : 31

Let me repeat: get a Slant Bar for your second razor. You'll be glad that you did, or at least 70% will be *very* glad, 23% will like it, and 7% of you will wonder why I recommended it: YMMV. Use a light touch with the Slant.

Whatever razor you get as a second razor, you should accept that you will have to "learn" it, much as you learned to shave with your first DE razor, though of course the learning time for the second razor is much shorter—sometimes just a single shave will do, sometimes a week or more before nicks stop altogether, generally somewhere around 3-4 shaves.

Understand, too, that a new razor may well have a different head geometry, which is why you have to learn it. One result of a different head geometry is that you'll have to experiment some with the angle: the new razor may require a shallower angle, for example. You may want to do a little blade exploration as well: your old best brand of blades may not work so well in the new razor. Judicious experimentation is always a good idea.

I believe that learning the second razor will be easier and go faster if you shave exclusively with the new razor until you once again are getting smooth, nick-free shaves with no razor burn. At that point you can probably switch back and forth between your new and old razor and your unconscious will make any technique adjustments for you.

I say again: your second razor should be a Slant Bar.

Whether to collect

Although most shavers begin DE shaving to save money—"The blades are so cheap! Look at much money I'll be saving in just a year!"—it would be disingenuous not to take notice that many find that shaving becomes a hobby and start spending on razors, brushes, shaving soaps and creams, aftershaves, and the like. While the supplies will ultimately be used (one hopes), a large collection of razors and brushes (and shelves on which to display them) can quickly run into money. (This is especially true of straight razors.)

Think about whether you desire—or can afford—to go into collecting. There's much to be said for viewing a razor and a brush as one views a hand-drill and a hammer: specialized tools to do a specific job. You pick one good razor, one good brush, and get on with it. You may want to upgrade the razor—for example, start with a Lord L6 and after the handle breaks, replace it with one of the Edwin Jagger DE8x series (or the Mühle equivalents), and perhaps ultimately get a Weber, selling off or giving away each razor as it is replaced, and follow a similar route for the brush.

Or you can set limits: three razors, three brushes, and that's it. Note, however, that this could be the beginning of a slippery slope. It does make sense, however, to have different razors of very different types for different jobs: for example, a Slant Bar for removing stubble easily, an Edwin Jagger for variety, and perhaps a Gillette Tech vintage razor, a mild shaver, for a polishing pass. And you might want a regular brush for home and also a travel brush, perhaps a Wee Scot or Omega 11047 or one of the Mühle travel brushes.

A larger collection can take on a life of its own, with the tail wagging the dog: the collection pushing the collector to extend it continually. Consider that any collection at some point must find a new home, and a large collection can be a challenge to dismantle. As in most of this book, I am writing from my direct personal experience, which currently includes downsizing for a move. I suggest that you carefully consider rigorous limits to collection size: a few—say, five— different razors and an equal number of brushes can offer a good variety that's nonetheless consistent with seeing razor and brush as tools, just as you might own a range of hammers—a tack hammer, a framing hammer, a ball-peen hammer, a mallet, and a sledgehammer—and still view (and use) the hammers as tools rather than collectible artifacts.

If you truly want to collect, consider collecting individual razor blades in their colorful paper wrappers. These come in a great variety—as you can see in your sampler pack—and offer a relatively inexpensive collecting venue. Moreover, razor blades require little space and are easy to store and transport, perhaps mounted in photograph albums with the plastic-wrapped pages.

I won't address supplies: those you can figure out (and use up). Although it's not actually collecting, I do suggest you try at least a shaving soap and a shaving cream, and it's worthwhile to get both a soap in a tub and a shave stick: if you don't explore some of the options, you will not learn what your own likes and dislikes are. But be careful even here: it's easier than you think to acquire a five- or ten-year supply of shaving soaps and creams.

With aftershaves, I think it's easier. You might want a few, of different types: a light fresh aftershave, a more musky aftershave, and perhaps a floral and a citrus... Well, maybe it's not so easy. But beware of getting too many. One good thing about shaving soaps, creams, and aftershaves: they're naturals for gifts, and with a little judicious hinting at the right times of the year, you can easily achieve a good selection.

Here are some suggestions regarding razors and brushes, which tend to be the big-ticket items: First, think about setting limits if you're inclined to collect, limiting either quantity or price or both. For example, if your interest is vintage Gillettes, you might decide that you will not spend more than $20 on a razor. This makes the hunt more difficult and a find more exciting. Or if your interest is brushes, you might decide that you will buy only old brushes for under $10 with the idea that you'll restore them, replacing the knot—probably a good idea in any case, since frequently the knot on old brushes is ratty and also difficult to sterilize if that's a concern. A nice sequence showing a brush restoration in detail can be seen on Wicked Edge[208].

Another approach might be to acquire one single representative of each type of razor or brush. For razors, perhaps a three-piece, a TTO, and an adjustable. Or you could go for six razors: those three types in an open-comb design and a straight-bar design. I, of course, believe that any set of razors should include a Slant Bar: it's an interesting razor, unique in its cutting action, and for most shaves extremely well. And speaking of unique razors, it's tempting to add an asymmetric razor to the mix: an unusual and intriguing design.

Another possibility is to focus on (say) the Gillette Super Speeds or the Gillette adjustables. Though either collection may have more different razors than you at first would think, at least you are focused on a single type of razor.

For brushes, you might first want to get one brush of each type: badger, boar, horsehair, and synthetic to experience their different qualities (thus exploring your own preferences) and get an idea of the range. If you get another brush of a type, you get rid of the one of that type you already had. Even if you throw in the hybrids—badger+boar, badger+horse, and boar+horse—that's just seven brushes: one for each day of the week.

Some unusual brush(es) might be included—for example, the tiny brushes: a Wee Scot in badger, an Omega 11047 for badger+boar, and a small horsehair and small boar brushes. Small badger brushes, though uncommon, are made by other manufacturers as well: I have one by Omega and I've seen photos of an absolutely tiny Plisson.

For both razors and brushes you can find stunning examples of custom craftsmanship. For example, Elite Razor and Rod Neep of Pens of the Forest offer some remarkable razors and brushes. These are unique—truly collector's items—but with custom creations, how do you decide when to stop? That's the danger. Moreover, fine items such as these tend to be expensive.

The idea of a "collection" is that it is not simply a bunch of stuff but instead a bunch of stuff with a definite structure that reflects a specific plan. Approaching your purchases with a plan that you've developed after some thought will help you know what you're not interested in (because it doesn't fit your collecting plan), and it also helps you to know when your collection is complete (if such a thing is possible).

FOURTEEN

Sources of the most common problems

PROBLEMS you encounter in shaving usually—though not always—have their source in one of the following areas. If you have some problem in your shave that doesn't seem to stem from the causes listed below, the shaving forums (see Appendix) are a good source of informed (albeit sometimes inconsistent) advice.

Hard Water

Hard water is a "hidden" problem because most shavers never consider water quality, and assume that their problems in making lather are due to their lack of skill. If a high-glycerin pre-shave soap doesn't add lubricity and produce a better shave, hard water is again the prime suspect. A distilled-water shave is easy to do and will show whether hard water *is* the problem, so if a pre-shave soap doesn't help your shave and/or getting a good lather is difficult, get distilled water and try it. If the shave is markedly better, use distilled water regularly.

Another common source of lather problems, particularly from soaps, is that the brush has not been loaded with enough soap. If your lather is mediocre, before trying distilled water (especially if the pre-shave soap does leave a lot of lubricity on your skin), make sure you're fully loading the brush. Brush the puck of soap *at length, briskly,* and *firmly* for 20-30 seconds (or until all large bubbles are gone and you see only fine-grained lather). Thus you continue brushing even after lather has started to form on the puck. Your initial focus is to load the brush fully with soap—you can work up the lather more on your beard, perhaps there adding a little water if it's needed (if the lather seems too dry).

Insufficient Prep

Your beard must be fully wetted to soften. Shave after showering, wash beard again at the sink with a pre-shave soap, and apply a good lather—dense and holding a substantial amount of water—to your wet beard. You can also try the hot towel treatment. Do **not** neglect prep of your neck shaving area.

One sign of insufficient preparation—and, in particular, of a lather that's too dry and/or a lathering process that's too brief—is that the blade seems dull, pulling and tugging at the beard instead of cutting smoothly and easily. It may be, of course, that the blade *is* dull, particularly if you've been putting off changing it. Or, if it's a new brand, it may be either a bad blade or a brand that doesn't work for you (or both, of course).

But if you have a brand of blade that's been working well for you, and suddenly it doesn't seem to be cutting, suspect the prep. Make sure the lather's wet enough, and spend a good amount of time with the brush, working the lather over and into your beard. Begin your shave with the softest part of your beard, leaving the toughest (the chin and upper lip) for last so that those whiskers have more time to soak in the lather and thus soften.

Wrong Blade for You

Blade selection is crucial. Novices focus on the razor, but the razor is just a device for holding the blade and presenting the edge at the correct angle to the stubble. Different people require different blades. Get a sampler pack so you can find the best blade for you. This step is absolutely essential if you want close and comfortable shaves. Don't skip it. And you *cannot* rely on recommendations from other shavers: one man's pebble is another man's pearl, and vice versa.

This idea is enormously difficult to grasp—if you have a terrible shave with a blade, it's hard to believe that others would actually *like* the blade, and if you have a wonderful shave, you want to recommend the blade to everyone. And yet it's true that *every* brand of blade has those who love it and those who hate it. Until you try the blade, you don't know into which group you fall.

Incorrect Blade Angle

Blade angle is absolutely critical. The blade should be *almost* parallel to the skin being shaved, so that the blade's edge strikes the stubble almost at a right angle as the blade slides over your skin. Generally speaking, keep the cap's edge—just behind the blade's edge—in contact with your skin. Focus on that and forget about the guard bar. Think of the blade as gliding along parallel to the skin, riding on a thin layer of lather.

Where the skin has a lot of curves (for example, jawline, neck, chin), you have to maneuver the razor a fair amount to keep the blade angle correct because the safety razor, unlike the cartridge razor, does not pivot. Making short strokes helps you stay focused on blade angle. Even with light pressure, if the angle's wrong, you'll nick or cut yourself.

Too Much Pressure

Shaving with a cartridge either requires or encourages pressure, so exerting too much pressure is a habit that cartridge shavers must unlearn.

Often the weight of the razor by itself is enough to cut the stubble. Hold the razor to minimize pressure—for example, by the balance point on the handle. When you rinse after the first pass, you'll feel quite a bit of stubble. This does **not** mean you should use more pressure—in single-blade shaving, you eliminate stubble by progressively reducing it over 2, 3, or 4 passes.

Keep the pressure light. Your face will thank you.

Ignoring Your Beard's Grain

It's vital that you know the direction of your beard's growth, since the sequence of passes is first *with* the grain, then *across* the grain, and then (if stubble is sufficiently reduced and you don't have to be concerned about razor bumps) *against* the grain. (If too much stubble remains for a comfortable against-the-grain pass, first shave across the grain the other way.)

Generally, the beard on your face will grow downward—but not always. I have a couple of patches where it grows more or less sideways. The grain on the neck can be anything, even whiskers growing in whorls, which is why good prep of the neck shaving area is so important. To find the grain, wait 12-24 hours after you've shaved, then rub your face and neck. The direction that's roughest is against the grain. You'll find the "roughest" direction is different on different parts of your face and neck. Use the interactive diagram[209] to map your grain.

Bathroom Too Loud

If your bathroom is not quiet—if, for example, water is running or the fan is on or you're listening to a radio—then you cannot hear the sounds of shaving. Shaving deaf, as it were, is like flying blind: it doesn't work well. You need auditory feedback to fine-tune the blade angle.

Setting an Adjustable Razor Too High

Some novices inexplicably dial their adjustable razor to the most aggressive settings—4, 5, or 6 on the Futur or Progress, or 8 or 9 on the Gillette Adjustable—and then find themselves staring in the mirror at their lacerated face. With adjustables, start with the *lowest* setting (1 on Futur or Progress, 2 or

3 on Gillette Adjustable), and advance the setting only as you must in order to get a good shave. As soon as you get a good shave, stop there. You want the lowest setting that works, not the highest setting you can stand. It's not a contest.

—

If you pay attention to these basic points, you'll enjoy your shaves. There will be a learning curve, as you make the transition from cognitive understanding to practiced skill, but you will at least know what you're trying for.

FIFTEEN

Where to get more information

NOW that you're at the end of this introductory book, you may well want to know more. Take a look at the on-line article[210] "Exploring the Science of Shaving" from the February 1957 issue of *Science and Mechanics*. The advice in the sidebar of that article, "10 Minutes to a Good Shave," is still right on target. A write-up on MSNBC[211] on how to get the perfect shave covers some of what's in this book.

The series of videos[212] by Mantic59 offers an introduction to and demonstration of many of the topics covered above. Betelgeux of Wicked_Edge also regularly posts shaving videos on his YouTube channel theshockwav. Geofatboy[213] also has an enthusiastic following for his shaving videos.

The wetshaving forums are a good source of information on new products and also offer invaluable advice to novices. You can post your own questions and receive in return a range of views and advice, which is all to the good: shaving solutions vary quite a bit from shaver to shaver, so knowing a range of solutions is useful. You must, of course, test proposed solutions to see whether someone else's solution will work for you.

One particular benefit of using the forums is that, when you describe a problem you're facing, you will often get responses from men who have faced (and solved) the identical problem, so you can profit from their direct experience. You will get better help if you provide a good description so that the advice you get is useful. Include at least the following:

- The brush you're using (brand and also the type of bristles)
- Which brand of shaving soap or shaving cream you use

- Whether you are using hard or soft water (or you don't know)
- Your prep procedure—whether you shave after showering, what pre-shave treatment(s) you do (if any), whether you use a hot towel
- The make and model of your razor
- The brand of blade and whether you have tried other brands
- The sequence of your passes and which passes you do (with, across, against the grain) and whether you've mapped your beard's grain
- The kind of problem you're having (nicks? rash? bumps?) and when it appears (during shave? right afterwards? an hour after? next day?)
- Where you live (which state/province and country?) to help with vendor recommendations—which state also gives an insight into whether water is likely to be hard

The reason for most of these is evident. The blade information is to determine whether you're simply using the brand that came with the razor (for example, Merkur blades), or whether you've done some exploration. By providing that information, you'll get much more helpful answers. If you don't provide the information, you will be asked for it anyway, so giving it at the start smooths the process.

Some manufacturers of shaving products offer samples (free or at low cost), which are quite useful. A sample is more than enough to test the fragrance and see whether you have any special sensitivity or allergic reactions. On ShaveMyFace you can find a comprehensive list[214] of sources of samples, and Garry's Sampler Shop (see Appendix) offers a good selection (and will consider requests, particularly for popular items).

Finally, the best source of information to improve your shave is likely to be your own experience and experiments and observations and reflection.

If you are wondering whether your lather is sufficiently wet—or too wet—the best course is to experiment: try using less water, then using more water, and see how it works for you.

If you are wondering whether a particular pre-shave you have really works, or whether it works better if you apply it before each pass, experiment. Shave a week with it, followed by a week without. Try a week of using it only before the first pass, followed by a week of using it before every pass. If a week's too long, try just two days.

Thoughtful experimentation and close observation of outcomes are, in shaving as in science and life in general, the most reliable source of knowledge.

Go now and experiment.

Appendix

Links are also available at **tinyurl.com/leisureguy5** in clickable form.

Forums

Art of Manliness Real-Shaving group – tinyurl.com/7bbx9ea
Badger & Blade –adgerandblade.com
Damn Fine Shave – damnfineshave.com
Pogonotomy - pogonotomy.com
Razor and Brush message board/sales board - tinyurl.com/2hj8db
RazorAndStone – razorandstone.com
Shave Bazaar (buy/sell/trade) – reddit.com/r/shave_bazaar
Shave Canada – shavecanada.ca
ShaveMyFace –shavemyface.com
Shave Nook – shavenook.com
Straight Razor Place –straightrazorplace.com
The Shave Den - theshaveden.com
The Shaving Room – theshavingroom.co.uk/forum
Wicked Edge - reddit.com/r/wicked_edge

Reference

Bruce on Shaving – bruceonshaving.com (many photos)
Gillette historical pricing strategies - tinyurl.com/3cjbgtj
Gillette Rockets - tinyurl.com/78qzjlr
Gillette date codes – gillettedatecodes.com
Mantic59's shaving videos - tinyurl.com/y2fx33
Mr-Razor.com tinyurl.com/c6whpw2 (in German: use Google Translate)
Museum of safety razors - tinyurl.com/3yzsm2
Schick Injectors - tinyurl.com/27vor9
Sharpologist – sharpologist.com
Shaving 101 – shaving101.com
Shaving information – shaveinfo.com
Shaving product samples - sampleshop.blogspot.com and
tinyurl.com/2gwu8c

Blade Sampler Packs

The vendors selling blade sampler packs as of this edition are:
- BestShave.net (in Turkey; free shipping for blade samplers)
- BullGoose Shaving Supplies (in the US)
- Connaught Shaving (in the UK)
- Details for Men (in the US)
- Em's Shave Place (in the US)
- Fendrihan (in Canada)
- Italian Barber (in Canada)
- Kinetic Blue (in Australia)
- Lee's Razors (in the US)
- Pureman.com.au (in Australia)
- Razor Blades & More (in the US)
- Razors Direct (in the US)
- Royal Shave (in the US)
- The Shave Den (in the US)
- Shave Nation (in the US)
- Shave Shed (in Australia)
- Shaving.ie (in Ireland)
- Shoebox Shaveshop (in the US)
- Straight Razor Designs (in the US)
- Total-Shave (in the Netherlands)
- Traditional Shaving Supplies (in Ireland)
- West Coast Shaving (in the US)
- Via Amazon.com: tinyurl.com/ycq3fb7
- Via eBay.com: tinyurl.com/6azkz5s

Vendors

Following is a list of on-line vendors for the wetshaving community. This list is volatile, as new vendors come on-line, so also check the supplemental post.

* = complete vendor (brushes, soaps, creams, razors, blades, aftershaves)

H = handmade shaving soap, creams, lotions, aftershaves, etc.

C = will accept calls from men seeking product advice

H **Al's Shaving Products** – alsshaving.com – contact form on the site – Exceptional shaving creams made by a straight-razor shaver initially for his own use. Try the 7-day pack of samples. He also makes aftershaves. The fragrances are excellent and he offers custom-fragranced shaving cream.

Appleton Barber Supply - tinyurl.com/7xy3j5u - 800-236-0456 Central Time - info@appletonbarbersupply.com - Primarily of interest for great selection of aftershaves (at link).

Art of Shaving - theartofshaving.com - 800-696-4999 Eastern Time - AOS shaving cream and soap and aftershave, Merkur. (Shave oil not recommended: too gummy). Soap and brushes excellent but expensive; limited range of DE shaving products.

Atkinson's - tinyurl.com/2dc6zy - info@atkinsonsofvancouver.com - 604-736-3368 800-803-0233 Pacific Time - Plisson brushes.

BadgerBrush.net – badgerbrush.net - This site offers attractive handcrafted shaving brushes and DE razors (with Edwin Jagger heads). A wide variety of woods are used. It also sells supplies for making your own brushes.

H* **Barclay Crocker** – barclaycrocker.com – sales@barclaycrocker.com – 800-536-1866 - Many brands of Bay Rum, Merkur, Proraso, Musgo Real (including Glyce Lime Oil pre-shave soap), Geo. F Trumper, Truefitt & Hill, Taylor of Old Bond St, Col Conk, Woods of Windsor, Shave Brushes & Mugs, Barclay Crocker Custom Scenting.

* **Best Grooming Tools** - bestgroomingtools.com - customerservice@bestgroomingtools.com - Selection includes Col. Conk, Dovo, Erasmic, D. R. Harris, Edwin Jagger, Merkur, Mühle, Musgo Real, Parker, Proraso, Simpson, Speick, Taylor of Old Bond Street, Valobra.

* **BestShave.net** – shop.bestshave.net – 90 0224 413 2710 – There's also a contact form on the Web site. Located in Bursa, Turkey. – Arko, Astra, Coll, Derby, Gibbs, Permasharp, Racer, Rapira, Shark, SuperMax. Free shipping on blades.

Blankety Blanks - tinyurl.com/rbwjd - djb@blankity-blanks.com - 512-263-8355 Central Time – Artisanal shaving brushes and supplies for making your own shaving brush (scroll down at link)

* **BM Vintage Shaving** – bmvintageshaving.com - sales@bmvintageshaving.com – 760-799-5539 Pacific Time - Col Conk, Derby, Dovo, Edwin Jagger, Gessato, Merkur, Taylor of Old Bond Street, Vulfix.

Bon Savon - tinyurl.com/2a67rx - info@bonsavon.com – 877-832-4635 Pacific Time - Provence Santé, Pre de Provence, Swedish Summer Soap, Lightfoot's Shaving Soap.

Bramble Berry – brambleberry.com - 877-627-7883 Pacific Time – Soapmaking supplies, including Melt & Pour Base for shaving soap: add your own fragrance.

* **Bull Goose Shaving Supplies** – bullgooseshaving.net - BullGoose@bullgooseshaving.net – Astra, Cyril R. Salter, Derby, Erasmic,

Feather, Lord, Merkur, Omega, Proraso, Shark, Simpson, Speick, Tabac, Taylor. Offers blade sampler packs.

Carbolic Soap Co. – tinyurl.com/yucvfb - Mitchell's Wool Fat Shaving Soap.

* **Classic Edge** – classicedge.ca – 416-574-1592 Eastern Time (Canada) - Has straight razors in addition to DE razors. Arko, Col. Conk, Derby, Dovo, D.R. Harris, Edwin Jagger, Feather, G.B. Kent, Lea, Merkur, Palmolive, Parker, Proraso, RazoRock.

CH* **Classic Shaving** – classicshaving.com – info@classicshaving.com – 760-288-4178 Pacific Time - Cremo Cream, Dovo, Feather, Merkur, Proraso, Rooney, Taylor of Old Bond Street, Thiers-Issard, Truefitt & Hill, Vulfix, Zowada.

H* **Connaught Shaving** – connaughtshaving.com - info@connaughtshaving.com - 07963 325842 - Carter & Bond, Derby, Gillette, Merkur, Parker, Proraso, Treet. Offers a blade sampler pack: tinyurl.com/yr36v2

The Copper Hat – thecopperhat.ca - They offer their own line of brushes, plus Parker and vintage safety razors, and products by Adam, Alpa, Pitralon, TrueShave, and Williams.

Crabtree & Evelyn - tinyurl.com/7n4xlgn - 800-272-2873 Eastern Time - Edwin Jagger brushes, C&E Shaving creams and soaps and aftershave.

* **Details for Men** – detailsformen.com - 888-680-2857 Eastern Time – contact@detailsformen.com – Art of Shaving, Derby, Feather, Gentlemens Refinery, Gillette, Musgo Real (including MR GLO), Pré de Provence, Proraso, Provence Santé, l'Occitane, Merkur, Mühle Pinsel, Speick, Valobra, Williamson, and others. Offers blade sampler packs.

eBarbershop – ebarbershop.com - sales@eBarbershop.com – Col. Conk, Crabtree & Evelyn, G. B. Kent, Merkur, Personna, Pinaud, Woods of Windsor.

eBay - Safety razors and blades – tinyurl.com/2hj626 At the link is a list of eBay offerings, including bulk-purchase Israeli and Derby blades, safety razors of all kinds, and the like. List sorted by newly listed, but can be resorted to find auctions ending soonest.

Elite Razor – eliterazor.com - robert.d.quinn@eliterazor.com – 404-918-2345 Central Time – Offers a wide variety of razors and brushes with handles custom-crafted of wood, stone, neo-resinate, or polycarbonate-covered snakeskin. Worth browsing for special gifts for traditional shavers. Available with Edwin Jagger head or Merkur Classic head.

H* **Em's Shave Place** – shaveplace.com and shaveinfo.com (the latter for shaving information and videos) – emily@shaveplace.com – Dovo, Em's (shaving soaps and creams, aftershaves, lotions), Geo. F. Trumper, Gold

Dachs, Merkur, Omega, Proraso, Simpson, Speick, Tabac, My Nik Is Sealed. Offers blade sample packs.

HC* **Enchante Online** - enchanteonline.com - enchantetx@sbcglobal.net - 888-220-2927 Central Time - Derby, D.R. Harris, Feather, Geo. F. Trumper, Israeli Personna, Merkur, Shavemaster, Taylor of Old Bond Street, Wilkinson.

* **The English Shaving Company** – theenglishshavingcompany.com - enquiries@theenglishshavingcompany.com - D.R. Harris, Edwin Jagger, Geo. F. Trumper, Proraso.

* **Esquires of Piccadilly** - esquires.com.au - sales@esquires.com.au - +618 9324 1101 Perth time - Dovo, Merkur, Taylor of Old Bond Street, Vulfix.*

Executive Shaving Company - executive-shaving.co.uk - Cyril R. Salter, Dovo, D.R. Harris, Edwin Jagger, Geo. F. Trumper, Rooney, Merkur, Taylor of Old Bond Street, Thiers Issard, Truefitt & Hill.

* **Fendrihan** – fendrihan.com - info@fendrihan.com - 905-230-1254 Eastern time. Col. Conk, Derby, D. R. Harris, Gold Dachs, J.M. Fraser, Merkur, Musgo Real, Simpson, Taylor of Old Bond Street, Valobra, Vulfix, Kent shaving soap (same as Mitchell's Wool Fat). Offers blade sampler packs.

Garry's Sample Shop – sampleshop.blogspot.com – A great resource for buying samplers of various shaving products (soaps, shaving creams, aftershaves, balms, and the like) so you can test them (for example, on your forearm) to be sure that you have no sensitivities that would preclude your use. Obviously, you also get a chance to check fragrance, lathering, etc.

G. B. Kent & Sons - tinyurl.com/4ftyn8 - +44(0)1442-232623 - vjp@kentbrushes.com - G.B. Kent shaving brushes (and hair brushes), Kent shaving cream and shaving soap (shaving soap is the same as Mitchell's Wool Fat Shaving Soap).

* **The Gentleman's Groom Room** – thegentlemansgroomroom.com - +44 (0) 1382 801504 – Arko, Arran Aromatics, Czech & Speake, Essence of Scotland, Floris, G.B. Kent, Geo. F. Trumper, Merkur, Mitchell's Wool Fat, Omega, Osma, Parker, Simpson, Taylor of Old Bond Street, Timor.

* **The Gentleman's Shop** - gentlemans-shop.com - sales@gentlemans-shop.com - 01488 683536 / 684363 (UK) - Art of Shaving, Castle Forbes, Dovo, D.R. Harris, Edwin Jagger, G.B. Kent, Geo. F. Trumper, Merkur, Rooney, Simpson, Taylor of Old Bond Street, Truefitt & Hill.

The Gentlemens Refinery – thegr.com – 866-444-7428 Mountain Time. Excellent shaving creams, aftershave balms, shave oil, shaving brushes.

* **Gifts and Care** – giftsandcare.com - contacto@giftsandcare.com - (+34) 96 3400 220 in Spain – Lots of horsehair brushes, including horsehair and boar

mix and horsehair and badger mix, in a range of grades. Also, Castle Forbes, Floïd, La Toja, Lea, Merkur, Myrsol, Proraso, Taylor of Old Bond Street. They also carry an extensive collection of makeup brushes.

H **Ginger's Garden** – tinyurl.com/85duy8w – Handmade "shaving-cream soap" that lathers abundantly and is available is a wide variety of fragrances. Also available is a glycerin soap. Soap comes as pucks, in tubs, or as shave sticks.

The Golden Nib – thegoldennib.com - Supplies for making your own brush: badger knots, handle blanks, razor heads, and more.

* **The Groomed Man** - thegroomedman.co.uk - 0844 8120465 - Cyril R. Salter, D.R. Harris, Derby, Dovo, Edwin Jagger, G.B. Kent, Merkur, Mühle, Simpsons, Taylor of Old Bond Street, Timor, Wilkinson

* **Highland Mens Care** – highlandmenscare.com - service@highlandmenscare.com – 877-284-1887 Eastern time – Acca Kappa, Anthony Logistics, Art of Shaving, Bluebeards Original, Castle Forbes, D.R. Harris & Co., Edwin Jagger, Feather, Gentlemens Refinery, Geo. F. Trumper, G.B. Kent, Lucky Tiger, Merkur, Musgo Real, Personna, Pre de Provence, Proraso, Royall Lyme, Taylor of Old Bond Street, Truefitt & Hill, Wilkinson Sword.

* **Himage** – himage.com.au - 1300 349 020 in South Melbourne - Astra, Castle Forbes, Coates, Col. Conk, Geo. F. Trumper, Mama Bear, Taylor of Old Bond Street, Truefitt & Hill, Cyril R. Salter, Derby, Dovo, Merkur, Proraso, Mitchell's Wool Fat, Mühle, Pashana, Simpsons, Vulfix, Semogue, Thayers

H **Honeybee Soaps** – honeybeesoaps.net - honeybeespa@att.net - Handmade shea butter shaving soaps and shave sticks, along with broad line of handmade creams, lotions, shampoos, and other toiletries. Wide variety of fragrances.

Ian Tang's Shaving Workshop - tinyurl.com/3pxa52w – Frank Shaving brushes: well-made but inexpensive badger shaving brushes.

iKon Razors – ikonrazors.com - Stainless iKon razors in a variety of designs, Feather blades, knobs for the Merkur Progress, and other offerings.

The Invisible Edge – theinvisibleedge.co.uk - Cutthroat razors and supplies in the UK.

* **Italian Barber** – italianbarber.com - support@italianbarber.com – 647-800-4622 Eastern time – Specializes in Italian shave products, but has wide range: Acca Kappa, Atkinson, Bolzano, Booster, Cella, Col. Conk, Cremo Cream, Feather, Geo. F. Trumper, iKon, J.M. Fraser, Lord, Merkur, Omega, Palmolive, Proraso, Rapira, Valobra, Wilkinson Sword.

H **Kell's Original** – kellsoriginal.com - dan.kell@kellsoriginal.com – A variety of excellent shaving soaps made with hemp oil, aloe vera, or a combination, in a variety of fragrances, including unscented. Sampler pucks available.

* **Kinetic Blue** - kineticblue.com.au - Astra, Dorco, Geo. F. Trumper, Merkur, Mühle Pinsel, Penhaligon, Truefitt & Hill. Blade sampler pack available.

KnifeCenter.com - tinyurl.com/7euhnnf – 800-338-6799
Altesse, Col. Conk, Dovo, Kent, Merkur, Omega, Parker, Pre de Provence, Thiers Issard.

* **Lee's Razors** – leesrazors.com – leesrazors@aol.com - 800-503-5001 Eastern Time - Col. Conk, Derby, Dovo, Feather, Geo. F. Trumper, Merkur, Mitchell's Wool Fat Shaving Soap, Musgo Real (including Glyce Lime Oil soap), Proraso, Simpson, Vulfix.

Lijun Brush - tinyurl.com/8xcv7dn – Inexpensive shaving brushes of reasonable quality from China.

London's Bathecary - shoplondons.com - 434-220-0540 Eastern Time - Caswell Massey, Floris London, Geo. F. Trumper, Lightfoot's, Mitchell's Wool Fat Shaving Soap, Penhaligon's, Taylor of Old Bond Street.

H **Mama Bear** - mamabearssoaps.com - sclark@core.com
Full line of handmade shaving soap, shave stick, shaving cream, aftershaves, along with regular soaps. Wide variety of fragrances. Also containers (make your own shave stick), alum block.

Mason Razor Works – masonrazorworks.com - Does restoration, repair, honing, scale replacement, and other services for straight razors.

* **Men's Biz** – mensbiz.com.au - 1300 784 789 – service@mensbiz.com.au – Astra, Col. Conk, Derby, Dovo, eShave, Feather, Geo. F. Trumper, Men-u, Merkur, Musgo Real, Personna, Proraso, Taylor of Old Bond Street,

men-ü - men-uusa.com - 800-987-6790 Central time – their own line: shaving creams and soaps, shaving brushes, and aftershaves. They offer an excellent synthetic-bristle brush.

* **Momentum Grooming** – momentumgrooming.com - shop@momentumgrooming.com - 604-689-4636; 1-877-886-4636 Pacific Time (Vancouver BC) - Merkur, Musgo Real, Proraso, True Gentleman, Truefitt & Hill

Moss Scuttle – sarabonnymanpottery.com - 902-657-3215 Atlantic Time - The famous Moss Scuttle along with a wide variety of pottery and hooked rugs.

* **Mühle-Pinsel** – muehle-shaving.com - info@muehle-shaving.com - German company. Baxter of California, D.R. Harris, Edwin Jagger, Geo. F. Trumper, Mühle-Pinsel, Proraso.

H **Mystic Water Soap for Men** – mystic4men.com - info@mysticwatersoap.com - 240-396-6831 Eastern Time - a good variety of excellent shaving soaps, tallow-based soaps using tallow from grass-fed beef raised locally in Maryland.

* **Nashville Knife Shop** – nashvilleknifeshop.com - info@nashvilleknifeshop.com – 812-988-9800 Central Time - Col. Conk, Cremo Cream, Derby, Dovo, D.R. Harris, Merkur, Proraso, Mühle-Pinsel.

Nancy Boy - nancyboy.com – contact@nancyboy.com - 888-746-2629 Pacific Time - Nancy Boy products, good for sensitive skin.

H **Nanny's Silly Soap Company** – nannyssillysoap.com – Many fragrances of handmade soft shaving soap.

H **New Forest Brushes** – newforestbrushes.blogspot.com – Handmade fine badger shaving brushes at very reasonable prices.

* **NkdMan.co.uk** – nkdman.co.uk – customer.support@nkdman.co.uk - Art of Shaving, Czech & Speake, Edwin Jagger, Merkur, Mühle, Proraso, Simpsons, Taylor of Old Bond Street, Truefitt & Hill

l'Occitane - tinyurl.com/6wjmrnw - 888-623-2880
Cade line of shaving soap, cream, shea butter aftershave balm.

H **Olivia Shaving Soaps** - tinyurl.com/2hxzey
Handmade shaving soaps and creams; Crema Sapone Cella.

Orient Outlet - stores.ebay.com/Orient-Outlet – An outlet for a Turkish store. Large selection of blades and Arko products.

Pacific Shaving Company - pacificshaving.com - Shaving oil, liquid styptic.

Penchetta Pen & Knife – www.penworks.us - 480-575-0729 – Primarily custom brushes and razors, but also stock Omega, Simpson, and Vulfix brushes and shaving creams and Parker razors.

Pens of the Forest - pensoftheforest.co.uk/shaving/ - Handmade shaving brushes and razors in unusual designs, with option of coin in base. Also sells fountain pens, penknives, etc.

* **The Portugal Online Shop** – theportugalonlineshop.com - info@theportugalonlineshop.com - portugalonlineshop@gmail.com - +351 962 774 286 Portugal - 444, Antiga Barbearia de Bairro, Ach Brito, Confiança, Musgo Real, Semogue. Many different pre-shave soaps available.

H **Prairie Creations** – prairie-creations.com – Handmade shaving soaps and creams, including shave sticks. The soaps are based on tallow or tallow combined with lanolin, with choices of scented, essential oils, or unscented.

* **Pureman** – pureman.com.au/mens-shave-care - info@pureman.com.au - (07) 3012 7990 in Brisbane - Astra, Baxter of California, Cella, Col. Conk, Derby,

eShave, Feather, Floris, Geo. F. Trumper, men-ü, Merkur, Personna, Proraso, Taylor of Old Bond Street, Truefitt & Hill.

CH* **QED** – qedusa.com - qed@quod.com
401-433-4045 Eastern Time - Castle Forbes, Cyril R. Salter, Geo. F. Trumper, Merkur, Musgo Real, Omega, QEDman (his own line of soaps and lotions), Proraso, Savile Row, Taylor of Old Bond Street, Truefitt & Hill.

H **Queen Charlotte Soaps, LLC** - queencharlottesoaps.com - info@queencharlottesoaps.com – Excellent handmade shaving soaps and shaving creams, along with shampoo bars, bath soaps, etc. The shaving soap contains tallow, palm oil, and coconut oil for a creamy lather; avocado, castor, and olive oil for skin conditioning; cocoa, shea butter, glycerin, and aloe vera extract for moisturizing; kaolin clay for a slickness; and natural vitamin E as an antioxidant.

Razor and Brush – mhbr.dk/razorandbrush - The site and store are gone, but the valuable content has been preserved.

* **Razor Blades and More** – razorbladesandmore.com – 323-362-6201 Pacific Time – Bluebeard, Cella, Coates, Col. Conk, Cyril R. Salter, Edwin Jagger, Erasmic, Feather, Floïd, Irisch Moos, La Toja, Lea, Malaspina Soap Factory, men-ü, Merkur, Mitchell's Wool Fat, Mühle, Musgo Real, Myrsol, Omega, Palmolive, Parker, Pinaud, Proraso, Speick, Tabac, Taylor of Old Bond Street, Valobra.

Razor Emporium – razoremporium.com – 602-885-2725 Mountain Time – an unusual site with an emphasis on vintage razors, both DE and straight, and vintage brushes. He also carries the Pils line, both razors and brushes. He offers a replating service for razors in gold, rhodium, nickel, silver, or other metals. Inquire for details.

Razors Direct – razorsdirect.com - 888-445-0224 Eastern Time - carries a good variety of razors (which this site calls "handles" rather than "razors"), and does offer a blade sampler pack. I've not ordered from them.

* **The Razor Shop** – therazorshop.com - 0422 953 284 Brisbane, Australia - Comoy, Dovo, King of shaves, Merkur, Otoko Organics, Proraso, Taylor of Old Bond Street, Shavemac, Vulfix, Truefitt & Hill, Zenith.

Restored Razors – restoredrazors.com - dave@restoredrazors.com - (0)7885 488189 – Does razor replating in nickel, silver, gold, or rhodium. Also sells vintage straight razors.

Retrorazor – retrorazor.com - chaddmbennett@retrorazor.com
Derby, Weishi, starter gift-packs, shaving workshops in Seattle

* **Royal Shave** – royalshave.com – info@royalshave.com - 800-801-0769 Pacific Time – Calani, Castle Forbes, Col. Conk, Edwin Jagger, Feather, Gold Dachs,

D.R. Harris, Hasslinger, G.B. Kent, Klar Kabinett, Merkur, Mitchells Wool Fat, Mühle, Parker, Pils, Plisson, Simpson, Speick, Taylor of Old Bond Street, Thater, Geo. F. Trumper, Truefitt & Hill, Vulfix.

* **SafetyRazors.co.uk** – safetyrazors.co.uk - info@safetyrazors.co.uk – +44 (0) 0845 009 0053 – Merkur, Taylor of Old Bond Street, Cyril R. Salter, Simpson. Also sells vintage razors. Contact for information about replating nickel-plated razors.

H **Saint Charles Shave** - saintcharlesshave.com sue@saintcharlesshave.com - Handmade shaving soaps, creams, aftershaves, lotions, eau de toilettes.

H **Scodioli** - etsy.com/shop/ScodioliCreative - Etsy vendor of handmade shaving soap, cologne, and other grooming supplies.

* **Sesto Sento** – sesto-sento.com - info@sesto-senso.com - 301-668-5018 - Castle Forbes, Geo. F. Trumper, Merkur, Musgo Real (including Glyce Lime-Oil Soap), Omega, Pashana, Proraso, QED Shave sticks, Savile Row brushes, Taylor of Old Bond Street, Truefitt & Hill, Vulfix shaving cream.

* **Shaveabuck** - shaveabuck.com – info@shaveabuck.com – 732-239-2607 Eastern time – A very broad selection including items hard to find in the US, at good prices. Includes Arko, Astra, Bea, Boots, De Vergulde Hand, Delong, Derby, Edwin Jagger, Erasmic, Feather, Frank, Godrej, James Bronnley, Kappus, G.B. Kent, Lavanda, Lea, Lightfoot's, Lord, Malizia, Merkur, Mitchell's Wool Fat, Mühle, Parker, Pitralon, Rapira, Sabi, Shark, Taylor of Old Bond Street, Timor, Treet, Valobra, Wars, Wilkinson

* **The Shave Butler** – theshavebutler.com – A Portuguese store; Bolzano, Col. Conk, Derby, Elios, Feather (blades and razors), Institut Karité, Iridium, Lavanda, Merkur, Mitchell's Wool Fat, Mühle, Musgo Real, O Melhor, Proraso, Semogue, Top Secret, Veleiro

The Shave Den Shop – theshavedenshop.com - part of The Shave Den Forum. Selection of shaving soaps and creams, both with fragrance oils and essential oils, along with aftershaves, colognes, and the like.

Shavemac - shavemac.com - info@shavemac.de - Dovo, Haslinger, Merkur, Olivesoap, Shavemac, Speick, Tabac, Weleda.

Shave Nation – shavenation.com - - 866-388-2088 Central Time - Cella, Col. Conk, Dovo, Edwin Jagger, Feather, Geo. F. Trumper, Mühle, Parker, Proraso, RazoRock, Taconic, Taylor of Old Bond Street, Tweezerman, Vitos. Has blade sampler packs. Lots of stuff for the straight-razor shaver.

* **The Shaver Shop** – shavershop.com – askus@shavershop.com – Col. Conk, Edwin Jagger, Geo. F. Trumper, HeadBlade, Merkur, Razor Guard, Tend Skin.

* **Shave-Shack.com.au** – shave-shack.com.au - enquiries@shave-shack.com.au - +61 (0)430 300 635 – The Otoko Organics shaving soap (under "Modern

Shaving") is remarkable. Also, Castle Forbes, Fitjar, Frank Shaving, Goodfella, Otoko, Proraso, Simpsons, Vulfix, Weishi.

* **Shave Shed** – theshaveshed.com.au - (03) 9005 6717 in Victoria, Australia - Col. Conk, Derby, Feather, Irisch Moos, Merkur, Mitchell's Wool Fat, Palmolive Proraso, Tabac, Taylor of Old Bond Street.

* **ShaveTools** – shavetools.com - 424-274-2838 Central Time - Astra, Cella, D.R. Harris, Gillette, Merkur, Omega, Parker, Proraso, Rapira, Taylor of Old Bond Street, Valobra, Vie-Long, Vulfix.

* **Shaving.ie** – shaving.ie – info@shaving.ie – 01 5240758 – Located in Ireland. Arko, Cella, Dovo, D.R. Harris, Edwin Jagger, Feather, Floïd, Geo. F. Trumper, Merkur, Mühle, Musgo Real, Omega, Parker, Pashana, Proraso, Semogue, Simpson, Speick, Tabac, Taylor of Old Bond Street, Timor, Vitos*

* **The Shaving Shack** – shaving-shack.com - enquiries@shaving-shack.com - 01752 898191 – Col. Conk, Cyril R. Salter, Dovo, D.R. Harris, G. B. Kent, Merkur, Mitchell's Wool Fat, Mühle, Musgo Real, Omega, Plisson, Simpson, Speick, Tabac, Taylor of Old Bond Street, Truefitt & Hill, Vulfix

Shaving Stuff - shavingstuff.com - Not a vendor, but a site that routinely reviews shaving equipment and supplies, from time to time finding things of interest to traditional wetshavers.

* **ShavingStyle** – shavingstyle.com – 647-773-1414 10:00 am - 8:00 pm Eastern time - Castle Forbes, Coates, Col. Conk, Cyril R. Salter, Dovo, Dubl Duck, Edwin Jagger, Goodfella, Merkur, Mühle, Omega, Proraso, RazoRock, Semogue, Simpsons, Tabac, Taylor of Old Bond Street, Vulfix, Wilkinson.

* **Shoebox Shaveshop** –shoeboxshaveshop.com - shoeboxshaveshop@yahoo.com – 786-200-2774 (between 8 a.m. and 8 p.m. Eastern Time) - Arko, Cella, Erasmic, Figaro, Fitness, Institut Karité, Lord, Mitchell's Wool Fat, Omega, Pre De Provence, PREP, Proraso, Speick, Tabac, Taylor of Old Bond Street, Treet, Weishi. Offers blade sampler packs.

* **Smallflower** – smallflower.com/men - Voice 800-252-0275 Central time - fax 773-989-8108 - Geo. F. Trumper, Mitchell's Wool Fat, Mühle Pinsel, Musgo Real (including Glyce Lime Oil pre-shave soap), Pre de Provence, Provence Santé, Proraso, Speick, Tabac. This is the on-line side of Merz Apothecary.

Straight Razor Designs – straightrazordesigns.com – service@straightrazordesigns.com – Baxter of California, Castle Forbes, D.R. Harris, Heirloom Razor, Maestro Livi, Merkur, Truefitt & Hill. Both straight and safety razor products.

Strop Shoppe – stropshoppe.com – Handmade shaving soaps by a biochemist from excellent ingredients (stearic acid, glycerin, coconut oil, palm oil, rice bran oil, and fragrance). Soaps lather quickly and abundantly. Also offers shaving brushes from Whipped Dog.

* **The Superior Shave** – thesuperiorshave.com - admin@thesuperiorshave.com – 904-482-1175 Eastern Time – Derby, Dovo, Feather, Merkur, Mühle (including travel brush), Omega, Parker, Proraso, Simpson, Thiers-Issard, Valobra, Vulfix. He seems to carry more Mühle products than other vendors.

Superlather – superlather.com - help@superlather.com - 727.483.5639 Eastern time – Alt Innsbruck, Erasmic, Floïd, Ingram, Irisch Moos, Noxzema, P.160, Palmolive, Pitralon, Proraso.

Total-Shave.nl - tinyurl.com/7y949t3 – This is the English-language storefront of a vendor in the Netherlands. Arko, Cella, Derby, Feather, Omega, Palmolive, Parker, Proraso, Sharp, Speick, Super-Max, Tabac, Vergulde Hand, Wilkinson

Tradere Razors – tradererazors.com - Offers an artisanal stainless steel open-comb razor and also the handle sold separately. Razors are machined and manufactured in the US.

* **Traditional Shaving Company** – traditionalshaving.co.uk - 0871 662 9683 (no orders by phone) - Astra, Colonel Conk, Crystal, Cyril R Salter, Derby, Edwin Jagger, Feather, Mama Bears Soaps, Merkur, Osma, Personna, Saint Charles Shave, Simpsons, Taylor of Old Bond Street, Truefitt and Hill.

* **Traditional Shaving Supplies** – traditionalshaving.com – info@traditionalshaving.com - +353 1 5240 758 in Dublin, Ireland. Acca Kappa, Astra, Cella, Coates, Edwin Jagger, G.B. Kent, Feather, La Toja, Merkur, Mitchells Wool Fat, Mühle, Omega, Semogue, Simpson, Speick, Sputnik, Tabac, Timor.

Tulumba - tinyurl.com/283vbt - info@tulumba.com 866-885-8622 Eastern Time - Arko, alum block.

C* **Vintage Blades LLC** - vintagebladesllc.com - jim@vintagebladesllc.com - 410-357-8055 Eastern Time - Col. Conk, D. R. Harris, Dovo, Floris London, Merkur, Rooney, Shavemac, Thayers, Taylor of Old Bond Street, Truefitt & Hill.

* **Vintage Scent** – vintagescent.com - A vendor in Portugal worth browsing for brands you won't find elsewhere: 444, Confianca, Floïd, La Toja, Lavanda, LEA, Semogue

Weber Razor – weberrazor.com - service@weberrazor.com - An artisanal solid stainless-steel three-piece razor, available in two models, one with head coated with "diamond-like carbon" and another with "ARC" (Advanced Razor Coating). They also sell the stainless handle separately.

C* **The Well Shaved Gentleman** - thewellshavedgentleman.com - 443-717-3969 Eastern Time - Sells excellent strops for straight razors.

* **West Coast Shaving** – westcoastshaving.com – contact@westcoastshaving.com – 877-710-6037 Pacific Time Cella, Gillette, Goodfella, Merkur, Mitchell, Proraso, Shavemac, Taylor of Old Bond Street, Valobra. Offers blade sampler packs.

* **Whipped Dog** – whippeddog.com - Secondhand straight razors of good steel restored to shaving shape. Feather Popular DE razor. Very good brushes at very good prices. Knots and other supplies to make your own razors. Free shipping. Good place for beginners to acquire a good starter kit at a low price. Also has a free introductory guide to straight-razor shaving (PDF – See tinyurl.com/836og9c). Offers blade sampler packs.

[1] Epicurus: See tinyurl.com/7kafxfj and (of course) the Wikipedia entry.

[2] Mihály Csíkszentmihályi: See tinyurl.com/a5f4s. Each person can find tasks appropriate for him or her that will promote flow: rock climbing, painting or drawing, gardening, cooking, playing a musical instrument, and the like. Csíkszentmihályi defined the term in his studies and in the fascinating book that emerged from them, *Flow: The Psychology of Optimal Experience* (tinyurl.com/ywzrea for inexpensive copies).

[3] Sharpologist article "Shaving-Tool Innovation and the Weber Razor": See tinyurl.com/6u98nm8 – and note also the article and (in particular) the comments to a *Harvard Business Review* blog post on Gillette strategy in India: tinyurl.com/bn77ohy

[4] Obsidian razor macrophotograph: See tinyurl.com/7uu93hm

[5] Obsidian razor shave: See tinyurl.com/6mzcz9y and tinyurl.com/7j9nmcq

[6] Miracle shaving device: See tinyurl.com/7r4qs3n

[7] Bruce Everiss low-cost high-luxury kit: See tinyurl.com/42telr2

[8] Whipped Dog beginner kit: See tinyurl.com/7majhlu

[9] Skin care: See tinyurl.com/2pttmv

[10] Gillette statement of cartridge life: See tinyurl.com/72dqnjk

[11] Andrew Webster shaving-cost Excel spreadsheet: See tinyurl.com/d8pj3xq

[12] Cognitive dissonance: See tinyurl.com/boyuz

[13] Ben Franklin was familiar with the effect if not the term. He decided to win over an opponent in the Pennsylvania state legislature:

> I did not … aim at gaining his favour by paying any servile respect to him but, after some time, took this other method. Having heard that he had in his library a certain very scarce and curious book I wrote a note to him expressing my desire of perusing that book and requesting he would do me the favour of lending it to me for a few days. He sent it immediately and I returned it in about a week with another note expressing strongly my sense of the favour. When we next met in the House he spoke to me (which he had never done before), and with great civility; and he ever after manifested a readiness to serve me on all occasions, so that we became great friends and our friendship continued to his death. This is another instance of the truth of an old maxim I had learned, which says, "He that has once done you a kindness will be more ready to do you another than he whom you yourself has obliged."

In terms of modern psychology, the opponent observed himself doing a favor for Franklin, a favor that Franklin framed as a great favor, and reduced his cognitive dissonance by deciding that he must like Franklin after all.

14 Life changes from new self-regard: See tinyurl.com/9yuyrev

15 Other personal-renewal notes: See tinyurl.com/7qko4ja and tinyurl.com/78y3z6f

16 Kamasori razors: See tinyurl.com/7mekms5

17 *The Art of the Straight-Razor Shave*: See tinyurl.com/ys9y5h (PDF) and tinyurl.com/6ptzfr9 (book)

18 *Straight Razor Shaving*: See tinyurl.com/7w7pz9s (PDF) and see also the discussion in this thread: tinyurl.com/83b8h99

19 Wilkinson technology: See tinyurl.com/2gce5h#218644

20 Intellectual-property law: See tinyurl.com/c7dgbte

21 Gillette strategy in India: tinyurl.com/bn77ohy

22 *Changing for Good*: See tinyurl.com/cslde8e

23 Shy/bold in animals: See tinyurl.com/blhmcl6

24 Explorer/settler brain chemistry: See tinyurl.com/cdlofqv

25 Report on revisiting Mach 3: Seee tinyurl.com/2ba4er#133588

26 "What was I thinking?": See tinyurl.com/2a4rm3

27 Returning to cartridges: See tinyurl.com/7mjs8ec

28 Women using DE razors: See tinyurl.com/7xcrdzy

29 eBay safety razors: See tinyurl.com/5n4l3g

30 For a wonderful account of the first-time experience, read what brderj and DEsquire say: See tinyurl.com/2aln4w.

31 *Getting to Yes*: inexpensive secondhand copies: See tinyurl.com/colwljd

32 *Predictably Irrational*: secondhand copies: See tinyurl.com/ckydhpm

33 Restoring old brush: A three-part series showing one restoration: Part 1: See tinyurl.com/7lr7xd3 Part 2: See tinyurl.com/6q9wrvb Part 3: See tinyurl.com/6tf3jy5

34 Wire-bending tool: See tinyurl.com/4455xy7

35 Videos by Mantic59: See tinyurl.com/y2fx33

36 Videos by betelgeux (theshockwav): See tinyurl.com/6tqdmyt

37 Mantic59's Advanced Shaving Techniques video: See tinyurl.com/2tzyeu

38 Interactive beard-map diagram: See tinyurl.com/7waok6b

39 Photosensitivity: See tinyurl.com/7nnvgqw

40 Potentially harmful cosmetic ingredients: See tinyurl.com/25jy9rq and tinyurl.com/6teu7x8 for two lists; a search for "harmful cosmetics ingredients"

will produce a plethora of lists—use your own judgment to determine the reliability of any particular list. Note also that skin types vary considerably.

[41] Tallow as plant product: See tinyurl.com/7c2a9x6

[42] Hair conditioners: See tinyurl.com/ytfhfn

[43] Ach. Brito Glyce Lime Glycerin soap: See tinyurl.com/dxyhmru

[44] Pre-shave soaps article: See tinyurl.com/7amxgov

[45] 100% glycerin: See tinyurl.com/7b8qe6p

[46] Pre-shave oil recipes: See thread at tinyurl.com/cx9czp2

[47] indiexsunrise shave oil recipe: See tinyurl.com/ceogrnq

[48] Softens the beard: What happens to the whisker in the presence of lather, water, and moist heat is complex, with "soften" being the common colloquial shorthand for the results of the process; see tinyurl.com/7jzfs2l I will use the word "soften" to describe how the beard becomes more amenable to cutting even though at a technical and microscope level the word is not accurate.

[49] Hydrosol: Herbal distillates are aqueous solutions or colloidal suspensions (hydrosols) of essential oils usually obtained by steam distillation from aromatic plants or herbs. These herbal distillates have uses as flavorings, medicine and in skin care. Herbal distillates go by many other names including floral waters, *hydrosols*, hydrolates, herbal waters, toilet waters, aqua vitae, and essential water. See also tinyurl.com/829uony

[50] Somewhat drier: See tinyurl.com/23cop2

[51] Synthetic bristles: See tinyurl.com/22r92w – Edwin Jagger synthetic brushes: See tinyurl.com/l3keno – Mühle synthetic brushes: See tinyurl.com/6uaqxwp

[52] Advantages of synthetic bristles: See tinyurl.com/296dbno

[53] Horsehair brush anthrax scare: See tinyurl.com/26hwnp8

[54] Suribachi bowl: See tinyurl.com/ykfzaav

[55] Semogue 2000: I suggest you avoid it, but see tinyurl.com/7ff3q3s

[56] Omega boar family: See tinyurl.com/7ca4leq

[57] Guide to boar brushes: See tinyurl.com/28kp67r

[58] Several grades: See tinyurl.com/23vwkc

[59] Made by hand: See tinyurl.com/2y4wev

[60] Clear differences: See tinyurl.com/yow8zh

[61] Vulfix brushes: See tinyurl.com/8bkbu

[62] Simpson brushes: See tinyurl.com/24ntes, tinyurl.com/ywt35u, and tinyurl.com/78s8zj9

[63] Gary Young on the Wee Scot: See tinyurl.com/6roacgv

[64] Rod Neep artisanal shaving brushes: See tinyurl.com/72j3fc4

65 Rooney brushes: See tinyurl.com/35b9ws and tinyurl.com/yrmm8k

66 Emilion, Victorian, and Thäter with hooked tips: See tinyurl.com/7b6v3me

67 Gary Young on hooked bristles: See tinyurl.com/7p4vyrv

68 Andrew's close-up photos of hooked tips: See tinyurl.com/7tpr4p9

69 Simpson measurements: See tinyurl.com/24kuln

70 Omega brushes: See tinyurl.com/yrdzbu

71 Omega brush measurements: See tinyurl.com/2c6pad

72 Kent brushes: See tinyurl.com/g8zyf (also has Rooney and Edwin Jagger
   brushes). The BK4 is the best size.

73 Bruce Everiss review of Morris & Forndran brushes: See tinyurl.com/3rxewcj

74 Bruce Everiss review of New Forest brushes: See tinyurl.com/3reovy9

75 Wooden-handled brushes: See tinyurl.com/22prko

76 Shaving brush innovations: See tinyurl.com/22xrfs

77 One video: See tinyurl.com/yvfjjf

78 Some nice accessories: See tinyurl.com/2bnqoe

79 Mühle travel brush: See tinyurl.com/2ayjrvg

80 Anatomy of hair shaft: See tinyurl.com/3elobn

81 Brush cleaning: See tinyurl.com/yvmfr6

82 Gold Dachs Shaving Brush cleaner: See tinyurl.com/3yrlw7p

83 M.A.C. brush cleaner: See tinyurl.com/8y8trf9

84 Moss Scuttle: See tinyurl.com/27ultr

85 Dr. Moss quotation: See tinyurl.com/ytfqz3

86 Georgetown Pottery: See tinyurl.com/74h43ux

87 Robert's Feats of Clay: See robertsfeatsofclay.com

88 Dirty Bird Pottery: See tinyurl.com/3s2twxf

89 Rival Little Dipper lathering bowl: See tinyurl.com/7qfzjzq

90 Air well: See tinyurl.com/cj2k3f

91 Water softener technology and options: See tinyurl.com/3e7p22g

92 Sunbeam Hot Shot: See tinyurl.com/yqxzng

93 Zojirushi hot-water dispenser: See tinyurl.com/2gkf6b

94 UtiliTEA kettle: See tinyurl.com/e226e

95 Surprising improvement from distilled water: See tinyurl.com/79ab5e6

96 Hard-water regions: See tinyurl.com/6qfu8bu

97 Using scuttle for distilled-water shave: See tinyurl.com/7eaas9g

98 J.M. Fraser's shaving cream: See tinyurl.com/6mxzd7v

99 High praise: See tinyurl.com/2zp35v

100 Nancy Boy shaving cream: See tinyurl.com/6r82q4o

[101] An illustrated guide: See tinyurl.com/29zlku

[102] Mitchell's Wool Fat Shaving Soap: See tinyurl.com/yucvfb

[103] Tabac shaving soap: See tinyurl.com/8xtryze

[104] Rivivage shaving soap: See tinyurl.com/6osa6j4

[105] Virgilio Valobra shaving soap: See tinyurl.com/2c6pat

[106] Bruce Everiss review of Otoko soap: See tinyurl.com/3epaps4

[107] Essence of Scotland shaving soaps: available from The Gentleman's Groom Room (UK) and Razor Emporium (US).

[108] Bramble Berry melt-and-pour shaving soap base: See tinyurl.com/7zbuxee

Also a Wicked_Edge thread: See tinyurl.com/7cakwdw

Another recipe, at About.com: See tinyurl.com/lxpw7w

[109] More information: See tinyurl.com/2cbkvo

[110] This excellent tutorial: See tinyurl.com/pylqk

[111] Video referenced above: See tinyurl.com/yvfjjf

[112] To make a shaving stick from any glycerin-based shaving soap: (This will *not* work with triple-milled soaps.) First, get a shaving stick container (e.g., from tinyurl.com/cc8ggc). Put the glycerin soap in a Pyrex measuring cup, and put that in a pan of hot water. Heat the pan of water over low heat until it's 150ºF, then turn off the burner and leave it for a while. (The soap takes a while to melt.) You may have to reheat the water, but don't go over 150º. (Patience.) While waiting for the soap to melt, turn the pusher of the container so that it's at the bottom. Do not lubricate the container—and in particular, do **not** use silicone grease—it will waterproof your brush and kill the lather. When the soap has melted, pour it into the container and wait until it's cooled. Voilà! Your own shaving stick. If it does not advance easily out of the container, put it briefly in the freezer and then try again.

[113] Superlather video: See tinyurl.com/2a2z7t

[114] StraightRazorPlace superlather tutorial: See tinyurl.com/7jqzm4u

[115] Gillette myth of giving away razors to sell blades: See tinyurl.com/3cjbgtj

[116] Microphotographs: See tinyurl.com/3mzl3t

[117] Blade reviews with photos: See tinyurl.com/lpz5lf

[118] Feather Blade Safe: See tinyurl.com/2ddz2k

[119] Pacific Handy Cutters blade bank: See tinyurl.com/7vtayuz

[120] If you're willing to undertake learning to use a straight razor, check out StraightRazorPlace.com and also *The Art of the Straight-Razor Shave,* by Chris Moss—see tinyurl.com/2c4zuz—and the introduction to straight-razor shaving by Larry of WhippedDog.com—see tinyurl.com/7w7pz9s

For straight razors—sharpened, honed, and ready to shave—and accessories and advice, contact Straight Razor Designs (see vendor list above).

For an excellent introduction to straights (with diagrams), see tinyurl.com/ybwjkt6 at StraightRazorPlace.com.

[121] Three types of razors: tinyurl.com/yqxeah

[122] Razor handles from Pens of the Forest: See tinyurl.com/7w4tgy5

[123] Edwin Jagger razor head: See tinyurl.com/cfsfcog

[124] Edwin Jagger razors: See tinyurl.com/76l4ztc

[125] Inadvertent blind comparison: See tinyurl.com/7grj9ks

[126] Whipped Dog beginner kit: See tinyurl.com/6o7xwh8

[127] Bruce Everiss and the three razor shave: See (in sequence) tinyurl.com/7woayos and tinyurl.com/7ner5zw and tinyurl.com/2fhcsne

[128] Slant Bar history: See tinyurl.com/6obtzkz

[129] Slant works well: See tinyurl.com/8yldz4t

[130] Gillette slide: See tinyurl.com/2tzyeu

[131] Loading Progress: See tinyurl.com/24cgdb

[132] This advice (Futur): See tinyurl.com/2dsrxe

[133] Vision user's manual: See tinyurl.com/2b4h5t

[134] Tradere razor review by mpperry: See tinyurl.com/72p48lr

[135] Diamond-Like Carbon: See tinyurl.com/2sd7h3

[136] Common Gillette razors: See tinyurl.com/2zq4yh

Also see these Super Speeds: tinyurl.com/393qsb6

[137] Dates of Gillette razors: See gillettedatecodes.com

[138] Fat Boy disassembly instructions: See tinyurl.com/3dy8k6

[139] Lady Gillette photos: See tinyurl.com/3m5ldg

[140] Wilkinson Sword Classic review by Bruce Everiss: See tinyurl.com/3p83y5x

[141] Eclipse Red Ring review by Bruce Everiss: See tinyurl.com/3orgqps

[142] Schick Injector: See tinyurl.com/ygf3mn

[143] GEM G-Bar: See tinyurl.com/26mh3z

[144] Schick various models: See tinyurl.com/27vor9

[145] Pella single-edged blades: See www.tedpella.com/dissect_html/dissect.htm#anchor1606431

[146] Ultrasonic cleaning: See tinyurl.com/dkm7hx

[147] Bleached Fat Boy: See tinyurl.com/7pqw4xx

[148] Art of Manliness on restoring razors: See tinyurl.com/25cf8zq

[149] Maas metal polish: See tinyurl.com/7h2htl4

[150] Holding the tip: See tinyurl.com/2955zd

[151] Pointed out angle: See tinyurl.com/yuz6p4

[152] Tiny travel razor: See tinyurl.com/yuuwxn

[153] A similar approach: See tinyurl.com/29sstk

[154] Useful diagram: See tinyurl.com/ynkb5o

[155] The basic 4-pass method: See tinyurl.com/2akgaq

[156] Advanced shaving techniques: See tinyurl.com/2y9ovh

[157] Hydrolast Finishing Balm: See tinyurl.com/3ktec2

[158] Total Shaving Solution: See www.totalshave.com

[159] All Natural Shaving Oil: See pacificshaving.com

[160] Kinexium ST Shaving Oil: See tinyurl.com/6bmbzc

[161] Gessato Pre-Shave Oil: See tinyurl.com/5b9srw

[162] Non-comedogenic chart: See tinyurl.com/555esn

[163] Natural 1 oz bottle: See tinyurl.com/4w8beb

[164] Cobalt blue 1 oz bottle: See tinyurl.com/4fbabt

[165] First Method video: See tinyurl.com/4llmby

[166] Method shaving supplies: See tinyurl.com/3ktec2

[167] Wikipedia article on alum: See tinyurl.com/3dfw2qz

[168] One woman notes: See tinyurl.com/yqx6vk

[169] Aluminum not hazardous: See tinyurl.com/otyolw and also this PDF: tinyurl.com/7vjoevx

[170] Cheapest price I've found for My Nik Is Sealed: See tinyurl.com/7zhg3op

[171] Proraso Styptic Gel: See tinyurl.com/7ecx6vs

[172] KDS Lab Liquid Styptic: See tinyurl.com/72bnye4

[173] Lengthy review: See tinyurl.com/35ekgm

[174] Mantic59 video on aftershaves: See tinyurl.com/3f9vmtx

[175] Skin problems with aftershave: See tinyurl.com/nmrcn3

[176] Variety of fragrances: See tinyurl.com/y8kw3o

[177] Sampler package: See tinyurl.com/265x8v

[178] Thayers Aftershave: See tinyurl.com/2c3vnd

[179] Booster's aftershaves: See tinyurl.com/28edcgy

[180] Proraso pre- and after-shave: See tinyurl.com/yr8kn5

[181] *The Emperor of Scent*: For inexpensive copies, see tinyurl.com/6red2p7

[182] Wikipedia perfume article: See tinyurl.com/hmrda

[183] Mild acne photos: See tinyurl.com/5yy46f

[184] Moderate acne: See tinyurl.com/4dw4sf

[185] Severe acne: See tinyurl.com/3old4v

[186] Sulfur-based compounds: See tinyurl.com/6ef7x6

[187] AcneNet: See tinyurl.com/498ksr

[188] Acne.org: See www.acne.org See also this post for additional tips that may be of help: tinyurl.com/6etgup

[189] Low comedogenicity: See tinyurl.com/crl2u4y

[190] Wicked_Edge acne reference post: See tinyurl.com/84lb6gs

[191] Mayo Clinic articles: See tinyurl.com/44ufoj

[192] *Anticancer: A New Way of Life*: See tinyurl.com/rdhruc

[193] Findings on sugar: See tinyurl.com/3rthjeg for informative article in *NY Times* and tinyurl.com/3fp83sb for an extremely informative talk.

[194] Pictures of razor bumps and rash: See tinyurl.com/3qg7bh

[195] Themba's technique: See the threads at tinyurl.com/yr5lz6 and tinyurl.com/5qbqpj (scroll down at both links)

[196] Innomed Lice Comb: Easily found with a Google search

[197] Moore Unique Razor Bump Tool: See tinyurl.com/d2k24k4

[198] Bump Fighter Razor: See tinyurl.com/59lm8f

[199] Barbicide: tinyurl.com/4pvmou

[200] Bump Fighter: See tinyurl.com/bvxyop5

Bump Patrol: See tinyurl.com/3rt6hu

Dermagen Skin Revival System: See dermagen.info

Elicina Biological Treatment: See tinyurl.com/4ampxj

Follique treatment: See follicareresearch.com/Men.php

High Time Bump Stopper Products: See tinyurl.com/d3ouatk

Moore Unique Products: See tinyurl.com/blwgclg

No Mo' Bumps Aftershave: See tinyurl.com/3uugej

Prince Reigns Gel: See tinyurl.com/4buq27

Smart Shave Products: See smartshave.com

Tend Skin: See tendskin.com

[201] Homemade version of Tend Skin: See tinyurl.com/63jsl3

[202] Eczema from shampoo: See tinyurl.com/lpxygf

[203] A beginner shaving kit: See tinyurl.com/2fao4t

[204] Low-cost high-luxury shave: See tinyurl.com/42telr2

[205] Whipped Dog beginner kit: See tinyurl.com/7majhlu

[206] Bump Fighter Razor: See tinyurl.com/59lm8f

[207] Poll on ShaveMyFace.com: See tinyurl.com/kn6vz7

[208] Brush restoration: Part 1 – Photo at tinyurl.com/7449ff8 and thread at tinyurl.com/7lr7xd3 Part 2 – Photo at tinyurl.com/88h98eu and thread at

tinyurl.com/6q9wrvb Part 3 – Photo at tinyurl.com/7q5ez7h and thread at tinyurl.com/6tf3jy5

[209] Interactive diagram: See tinyurl.com/7waok6b

[210] "Exploring the Science of Shaving": See tinyurl.com/cb92ae

[211] Write-up on MSNBC: See tinyurl.com/48evm

[212] Mantic59's series of videos: See tinyurl.com/y2fx33

[213] Geofatboy shaving videos: See tinyurl.com/7lfr9mp

[214] A comprehensive list: See tinyurl.com/2gwu8c

Made in the USA
Lexington, KY
29 July 2013